Backs Against the Wall

Backs Against the Wall: Battered Women's Resistance Strategies tackles several controversial aspects involved with intimate partner violence (IPV)—namely the approaches many victims use when resisting their oppressors. This sensitive and sensible feminist perspective concerning battered women's use of different resistance strategies, and the reasons why they use them, also focuses on ways to support victims through intervention and prevention strategies. Leading experts provide current research, revealing viewpoints, and convincing assertions about the victims of IPV.

This book powerfully refutes the sweeping assertions made by today's antifeminist-based mindset that women are as violent as men in cases of IPV perpetration. This insightful source provides strong evidence of the different resistance strategies that battered women use in response to multiple oppressions, including IPV, in the case against the gender parity argument—that may very well be politically motivated. The text provides extensive references and several figures and tables to clearly present data.

This book is a valuable resource for activists, educators, students, health providers, justice system workers, advocates, and researchers.

This book was published as a special issue of the *Journal of Aggression, Maltreatment and Trauma*.

Kathy A. McCloskey is Associate Professor at the University of Hartford, Graduate Institute of Professional Psychology in Hartford, CT. Her specialties include domestic violence, trauma, forensic populations, and the training of doctoral-level clinical psychologists.

Marilyn Sitaker is Section Epidemiologist at the Washington State Department of Health in Olympia, WA, where she is responsible for surveillance and evaluation of policy and environmental interventions to reduce the prevalence of obesity and obesity-related chronic diseases.

Backs Against the Wall

Battered Women's Resistance Strategies

Edited by Kathy A. McCloskey and Marilyn H. Sitaker

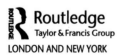

Routledge
Taylor & Francis Group
LONDON AND NEW YORK

First published 2009 by Routledge
2 Park Square, Milton Park, Abingdon, Oxon, OX14 4RN

Simultaneously published in the USA and Canada
by Routledge
270 Madison Avenue, New York, NY 10016

Routledge is an imprint of the Taylor & Francis Group, an informa business

© 2009 Edited by Kathy A. McCloskey and Marilyn H. Sitaker

Typeset in Times by Value Chain, India
Printed and bound in the United States of America on acid-free paper by IBT Global

British Library Cataloguing in Publication Data
A catalogue record for this book is available from the British Library

ISBN 10: 0-7890-3583-9 (h/b)
ISBN 10: 0-7890-3584-7 (p/b)
ISBN 13: 978-0-7890-3583-7 (h/b)
ISBN 13: 978-0-7890-3584-4 (p/b)

CONTENTS

ABOUT THE CONTRIBUTORS

Margaret E. Bentley is Professor of Nutrition and Associate Dean for Global Health at the University of North Carolina–Chapel Hill.

David Celentano is Professor and Director of the Infectious Diseases Epidemiology program at the Johns Hopkins University Bloomberg School of Public Health.

Dana-Ain Davis is former Assistant Professor of Anthropology at Purchase College, State University of New York. She is now Assistant Professor and Associate Chair for Worker Education at the Queens College Worker Education Extension Center in New York. Her research focuses on how people "live" out policy. She conducts research in both the United States and Namibia.

Donna Gardner, MA, MSW, was the Clinical Program Director for many years at Artemis Center for Alternatives to Domestic Violence in Dayton, OH. She received an MA in Public Policy and Management and an MSW from the Ohio State University. She is independently licensed as a social worker in the state of Ohio. Prior to working at Artemis, she provided therapy at a community mental health center and worked at a rural domestic violence shelter. For over a decade, she provided clinical supervision to victim advocates and child therapists. She implemented various projects, including the Montgomery County Domestic Violence Hotline and the Women Who Resort to Violence group. She has also trained police officers, prosecutors, physicians, victim advocates, and other professionals on issues concerning intimate partner violence. She currently resides is Florida and continues to consult with others within the field of domestic violence

Vivian F. Go is Assistant Professor in the Epidemiology Department at the Johns Hopkins University Bloomberg School of Public Health.

Sethulakshmi C. Johnson is a social worker currently working as the Ethnography Coordinator at the YRG CARE-Community Research Facility, Chennai, India.

Kathy A. McCloskey, PhD, PsyD, ABPP, is Associate Professor at the University of Hartford Graduate Institute of Professional Psychology in Hartford, CT. Her specialties include domestic violence, trauma, forensic populations, and the training of doctoral-level clinical psychologists.

Anne O'Dell is a retired Detective Sergeant from the San Diego Police Department, where she worked for 20 years. She is currently the Training Director for STOPDV in Poway, California. She is also an Adjunct Professor for the National College of District Attorneys, the California District Attorneys Association, and a Visiting Professor for Harvard University in Boston. She is a Consultant for the U.S. National Institute of Justice and the Department of Justice, as well as the Domestic Abuse Intervention Project of Duluth, MN.

Subadra Panchanadeswaran is currently an Assistant Professor at the Adelphi University School of Social Work, and previously served as a Research Associate at the Johns Hophins University Bloomberg School at Public Health. Her research interests include domestic violence, health effects of abuse and trauma on Immigrant women, and HIV/AIDS. She is a trained social worker with international work and research experience with communities and abuse survivers.

Mekha Rajan is a recant doctoral graduate of the University of Hartford Graduate Institute of Professional Psychology. She is also an affiliate of the American Psychological Association, Connecticut Psychological Association, and the Association for Women in Psychology. Her research interests include issues concerning domestic violence and issues involving South Asian Americans. Her contribution here is a further extension of a dissertation completed in partial fulfillment of the requirements for the degree of Doctor of Psychology.

Marilyn Sitaker is the Section Epidemiologist at the Washington State Department of Health in Olympia, WA, where she is responsible for surveillance and evaluation of policy and environmental interventions to reduce the prevalence of obesity and obesity-related chronic diseases. Prior to her work at the WSDOH, she was a Co-Investigator on the Community Partnerships Project and an Epidemiologist with the Intimate Partner Violence Surveillance Project at the University of Kentucky Injury Prevention and Research Center.

Sudha Sivaram is Research Faculty Member in the Department of Epidemiology at the Johns Hopkins School of Hygiene and Public Health.

Suniti Solomon is Director of YRG CARE, Chennai, India.

A. K. Srikrishnan is a Study Manager employed with YRG CARE, Chennai, India.

CarolynM.West is Associate Professor of Psychology and the Bartley Dobb Professor for the Study and Prevention of Violence in the Interdisciplinary Arts and Science Program at theUniversity of Washington, Tacoma. She is an award-winning author and Fellow of the American Psychological Association. Dr.West writes, trains, consults, and lectures internationally on interper-sonal violence and sexual assault. She is the author of numerous book chapters and journal articles, and is editor/ contributor of *Violence in the Lives of Black Women: Battered, Black, and Blue*, which was published by Haworth Press in 2002.

Prologue: Introduction and Overview to Special Issue

EDITORS

Kathy A. McCloskey

University of Hartford

Marilyn Sitaker

Washington State Department of Health

Editor Bios:

Kathy A. McCloskey, Ph.D. (Columbia Pacific), Psy. D. (Wright State University), Diplomat of the American Board of Professional Psychology in Clinical Psychology (ABPP), is an Associate Professor at the University of Hartford Graduate Institute of Professional Psychology in Hartford, CT. Her specialties include domestic violence, trauma, forensic populations, and the training of doctoral-level clinical psychologists.

Marilyn Sitaker: Ms. Sitaker is the Section Epidemiologist at the Washington State Department of Health in Olympia, WA, where she is responsible for surveillance and evaluation of policy and environmental interventions to reduce the prevalence of obesity and obesity-related chronic diseases. Prior to her work at the WSDOH she was a Co-Investigator on the Community Partnerships Project and an Epidemiologist with the Intimate Partner Violence Surveillance Project at the University of Kentucky Injury Prevention and Research Center.

Prologue: Introduction and Overview

When we first discussed putting this group of papers together back in 2002, we were aware of the increasing rates of battered women arrested for intimate partner violence (IPV) and wanted to somehow respond in a helpful way. We were also aware of the increasingly strident tone amongst some academicians and other social science researchers who insisted gender parity in IPV perpetration ("gender symmetry") was a truly serious public health problem. We were also aware that some were communicating, at least indirectly, that arrest rates were finally beginning to reflect what their research results had suggested all along – women are violent like men in heterosexual relationships – which could potentially negatively impact an already dwindling funding stream.

The first editor (McCloskey), the academic of the two, had attended a well-known international research conference in California and presented a paper there concerning sexual assault gender asymmetry data. Her co-presenters in that particular session were men who insisted that male sexual assault victimization rates are on a par with female rates overall and implicitly asserted that such information was being kept from the public, even though they could produce no evidence of either rates or a cover-up. These co-presenters were also observed by the first author repeatedly coming together with a handful of other men in the conference hotel hallways during and after presentation sessions where they conferred and then again fanned out. Every man in this group was a presenter, and every man in the group insisted that women and men are equal in their proclivity to both perpetrate and be victimized by violence in all forms. Most disturbingly, the first editor observed one of these men verbally accost a female colleague and publicly berate her during a particular lunch break concerning her refusal to agree that men are as victimized as women. When this colleague brought her concerns to the conference organizer, they were downplayed and dismissed.

The second editor (Sitaker), a public health expert, had by no means remained unaffected by the current state of affairs. She couldn't help but notice that somehow the IPV academic research field as a whole remained seemingly unaware of both the crucial measurement issues and available culturally-embedded information that directly impacted men's and women's victimization and perpetration. After all the years and all the volumes of public health research depicting men's behavior as the main health concern vis à vis violence, the second editor was amazed at the increasingly evident detour the IPV research field was taking in just the opposite direction.

Given our experiences, we had to do something. Between the two of us, in 2003 we contacted and recruited the present authors as collaborators for the book you are about to read. The two editors also provided the "book-end" manuscripts. Since our decision back in 2003 we have seen special editions concerning women's use of IPV published in five journals (*Journal of Offender Rehabilitation, Psychology of Women Quarterly, Sex Roles, Violence Against Women*, and *Violence & Victims*). Our present effort thus represents the sixth effort in a long line of publications appearing in the last few years concerning women's IPV. Obviously, this is quite the hot topic at the moment. The tone and stance of the articles in the journals listed above range from an understanding of the contextual and cultural issues surrounding women's IPV that refutes gender symmetry (e.g., M.A. Dutton & Goodman, 2005), to flat assertions that females are as abusive as males in intimate relationships (D. G. Dutton, Nicholls, & Spidel, 2005). To be quite clear, our special issue constitutes a feminist discussion of battered women's use of different resistance strategies of which violence is only one.

The first chapter in this special edition is by one of the editors (McCloskey), and provides an overview of the present controversy surrounding gender symmetry outlined above. She asserts that to truly understand women's use of IPV, it is crucial that researchers incorporate the effects of multiple oppressions women face within the context of predominantly male offending across different types of violent criminal categories. Furthermore, she states that we must integrate findings from both objective and subjective IPV research methods that will require elevating subjective approaches to the same status as objective methods, and that the on-going patterns of coercion, power, and control within our definitions of IPV need to be central. She presents an integrated research approach in the hopes of reducing or stopping the diversion of much-needed resources toward the so-called gender symmetry debate, and to curb any further injustices against women as a result.

The second chapter provides an overview of recent changes in the criminal justice response to IPV (specifically the adoption of preferred/ mandatory arrest policies) that are related to the current increase in women's IPV arrests (Rajan & McCloskey). A review of the recent forensic-related research since the advent of these changes suggests that arrests of women have increased overall by about 25–35%, while only about 1–7% of all IPV arrests are of actual female primary batterers. The authors suggest this is obvious evidence that victims are being arrested in larger numbers than ever before, and discuss some of the factors that may contribute to officers arresting not only primary batterers but victims as well. They also note the negative implications of errant victim arrests including legal, financial, employment, and familial repercussions.

O'Dell, a retired police officer, provides the third chapter that deals with the varied and complex reasons that police falsely arrest victims at the IPV scene. She suggests such reasons include the patriarchal/ paramilitary structure of police agencies, the staffing patterns of these agencies, and the inappropriate and inadequate training of officers. Her contribution presents real-life examples of cases where police arrested victims, and why these arrests occurred. She also includes thorough and detailed suggestions for how police agencies can minimize these illegal arrests within their jurisdictions.

In the fourth chapter, a long-time victim's advocate, Gardner, provides an overview of many of the ethical quandaries found when providing court-ordered services within an advocacy center to victims arrested for IPV. While the recent influx of victims mandated for batterer treatment raises many more questions than can currently be answered, she nevertheless presents suggestions for how to couch such ethical issues as well as provide effective advocacy in the face of such injustices. In addition, she provides a categorization that can aid in the identification of the different forms that women's violent resistance to gender-related oppression can take; this categorization can then be used to tailor mandated interventions accordingly.

A battered Black woman's first-person account of being falsely arrested is recounted in the fifth chapter (West) in order to examine the experiences of Black victim–defendants through narrative methodology. By illustrating how multiple intersecting oppressions negatively impacted one battered woman and resulted in her false arrest, the author makes a strong case for the presence of "bidirectional asymmetric violence" between heterosexual intimate partners. While the author asserts that violence is but only one strategy that battered women use in resisting their own abuse, she shows how such resistance may increase the chance of arrest. She follows this with an exploration of possible factors that may contribute to Black women's overrepresentation in the legal system, including the enactment of mandatory arrest laws. Finally, she offers strategies for advocacy and intervention with Black victim–defendants.

The sixth chapter is contributed by Davis who examines IPV through the lens of multiple contexts, in this case women's poverty and race/ ethnicity. She reveals that violence by women is not the only way that women resist the violence in their personal lives. She uses an ethnographic approach that utilizes battered women's survival stories. This approach reveals four different strategies, often varying by race, that battered women in poverty deploy in their protective trajectory. Her results also highlight the alternative resistance strategies women use to overcome multiple structural barriers (including poverty and IPV) present in their lives.

The seventh chapter by Panchanadeswaran and colleagues further extends our cross-cultural knowledge and understanding of alternative resistance strategies that women use in the face of IPV and poverty. She and colleagues use the *Theory of Gender and Power* to examine women's vulnerability to HIV infection in India. In order to further understand the vulnerability of female sex workers and married women in the context of poverty as well as violence within their sexual relationships with either clients or marriage partners, these authors also use an ethnographic approach. Their results highlight women's vulnerability to HIV infection stemming from partner violence, alcohol use, poverty, dangers of sex work environments, and the tacit acceptance of cultural/gender norms. Not surprisingly, violent male sexual partners emerge as an important barrier to the initiation and execution of successful safe sex negotiation with both male sex clients and marriage partners. However, these authors note the range of strategies women used to resist the violence and to negotiate safe sex practices, of which their own violent behavior was only one.

The eighth and final chapter is by the second editor (Sitaker). She ends the present volume by first describing the multiple factors associated with intimate partner violence (IPV) using the social-ecological framework developed by Heise. She uses this framework to categorize research findings from multiple disciplines according to the level of social organization at which they operate. She then provides a thorough and detailed review of evidence-based strategies according to both the sphere of social influence found in Heise's model and their place on the prevention continuum (primary versus secondary prevention). Throughout this integrated review, she also notes possible effects of risk factors and intervention strategies on women's use of IPV, particularly battered women's use of violence.

In summary, we wish to reiterate that our present effort is a feminist one intended to counter many of the more strident voices within our field that insist upon the "reality" of gender symmetry concerning IPV perpetration. We hope that you'll agree we've provided strong evidence of the different resistance strategies battered women use in response to multiple oppressions, including IPV, that refute the sweeping assertions of gender parity. Perhaps Brush (2005) best sums up our motivations behind compiling these manuscripts:

> Feminist researchers need to be vigilant about countering the ways anti-feminist pundits and policy-makers take findings out of context, extrapolate inappropriately, and misuse insights about the complexities of lived experience to undermine precarious public support for battered women and shelter funding ... a focus on women's aggression and violence can take the emphasis off the combination of gendered structure and agency behind two salient facts: most violence and aggression in most contexts are directed by men at other men, and women's risk for violent victimization is highest in the context of heterosexual couples ... the leap from finding that women aggress in a significant proportion of couples to an assumption of "gender symmetry" and from there to a "battered husband syndrome" which requires a response at the expense of services for battered women is politically motivated ... it is a frustrating reality that a research focus on women's aggression and violence can inadvertently fuel threats to funding and services to battered women, especially when anti-feminism is paired with conservative attacks on social provision. (p. 871).

Our thoughts exactly.

REFERENCE

Brush, L. D. (2005). Philosophical and political issues in research on women's violence and aggression. *Sex Roles: A Journal of Research*, 52(11–12), 867–874.

Dutton, D. G., Nicholls, T. L., & Spidel, A. (2005). Female perpetrators of intimate abuse. *Journal of Offender Rehabilitation*, 41(4), 1–31.

Dutton, M. A. & Goodman, L. A. (2005). Coercion in intimate partner violence: Toward a new conceptualization. *Sex Roles*, 52(11-12), 743–757.

Are Half of All IPV Perpetrators Women? Putting Context Back into the Intimate Partner Violence Research Field

Kathy A. McCloskey

In 2002, Watts and Zimmerman published a review article in the *Lancet* that highlights the global scope and magnitude of violence against women. These authors discuss the most common and severe forms of violence against women worldwide, with intimate partner violence (IPV) ranked alongside widespread religious and political oppression, forced marriage, the prostitution, trafficking, and debt bondage of women and girls, exploitation of women's labor, denial of reproductive agency resulting in forced pregnancy and birth, female infanticide, sex-selective abortion, abandonment of elderly females, and rape during war. They also state that perpetrators most commonly include spouses/intimate partners, parents of both genders, neighbors and other community members, and men in positions of power (business and/or religious leaders, politicians, etc.). Perhaps most strikingly, they assert that violent and oppressive acts against women are not isolated out-of-the-ordinary incidents but instead are part of the global social fabric as evidenced by ongoing and long-term cultural and institutional patterns. Their conclusions are two-fold: (a) because of the sensitivity of the issue and the invisibility of violence against women due to its wide-scale integration into prevailing global social norms, violence against women is grossly under-recognized and under-reported, and (b) its prevalence suggests that millions of women and their children are experiencing some form of violence at any given time, or at least living with its consequences (Watts & Zimmerman, 2002). This is true whether referring to under-developed and economically poor countries or the more technologically advanced, richer countries. The U.S. is no exception.

7

It is still common for many domestic violence researchers within the U.S. to overlook the deeply ingrained cultural and structural violence against women. The continuing plaintive question concerning battered women, "Why doesn't she just leave?" (Anderson et al., 2003), as well as the recent controversies within the IPV field over so-called "gender symmetry" or "mutual combat" between heterosexual partners (e.g., Johnson, 1995; Straus, 2006), underscore this state of affairs. At the beginning of the new millennia within the U.S., a cursory examination of our overall cultural discourse suggests we are dealing with a striking polarity in moral, spiritual, political, and religious beliefs coupled with a movement toward blaming those who are still actively oppressed by our social institutions. Individuals unjustly blamed for our current social ills include those in oppressed groups such as women, children, and adolescents; the poor; people of color; recent immigrants; and religious minorities (among others), especially when they actively resist their own oppression.

In the spirit of two feminist classics, Rianne Eisler's (1987) *The Chalice and the Blade: Our History, Our Future* and Susan Faludi's (1991) *Backlash: The Undeclared War Against Women*, it seems important to acknowledge that at this point in time we are again within a cyclical period of holding women accountable for their own victimization, especially as they are being blamed for their resistance within oppressive and violent intimate heterosexual relationships. As evidence for this, we find ourselves revisiting the issue of women's use of violence in general and IPV in particular. However, without a contextual lens to help us understand the current increase in attention to women's violence, those of us within the domestic violence field are just as susceptible to backlash forces as anyone else. As Chesney-Lind and Pasko (2004) write concerning the history of women's crime:

> . . . . research on the history of women's offenses, particularly women's violence, is a valuable resource for its information on the level and character of women's crime and as a way to understand the relationship between women's crime and women's lives. Whenever a woman commits murder, particularly if she is accused of murdering a family member, people immediately ask, "How could she do that?" Given the enormous costs of being born female, that may well be the wrong question . . . . the real question is why so few women resort to violence in the face of such horrendous victimization–even to save their lives . . . . in fact, women murderers . . . are interesting precisely because of their rarity. The large number of women arrested for trivial property and morals of-

fenses, coupled with the virtual absence of women from those arrested for serious property crimes and violent crimes, provides clear evidence that women's crime parallels their assigned role in the rest of society . . . (pp. 97-98)

Yet within the field of domestic violence research, we seem to be revisiting the issue of women's IPV in an ahistorical way, often ignoring the lessons of the past. Not only do we tend to ignore such lessons, we insist on taking the phenomenon of women's violence within intimate relationships out of its immediate cultural embeddedness. By doing so, some researchers whose harmful viewpoints and methods were once discounted due to poor overall construct validity now have an open arena to republish old chestnuts that assert there is an equal amount of IPV between men and women, and even to suggest there is an active "suppression of evidence on female perpetration by both researchers and agencies" (Straus, 2006, p. 1086). This is a sad state of affairs. One would hope that within the U.S. at the beginning of the 21st century, this fight would not have to be fought again. Unfortunately, such is not the case, and it is therefore time to insist we put the social context surrounding women's use of IPV back into the equation.

Re-Contextualizing Measurement Issues

Given the short review above concerning women's oppression, it seems that no one would believe the assertion that women as a whole are violent like men either inside or outside the home. Such a belief would have to be held in isolation from other knowledge bases. In order to overcome such an isolated and erroneous understanding of IPV, the following section shows the importance of starting large and then zooming in to the individuals involved (see Figure 1). Starting large (the top level) entails two steps: (a) re-embedding women's IPV within the multiple overarching forms of social oppression, and (b) then comparing gender-based knowledge across different domains of violent and criminal behavior. The next step (the middle level) entails focusing on IPV proper, while incorporating multiple measurement techniques in order to fully understand the phenomenon (not to mention insuring construct validity). The third and final step (the individual level) entails zeroing in on those individuals within relationships where IPV is present and evaluating not simply acts of violence at one point in time, but instead including ongoing patterns of coercion, power, and control.

FIGURE 1. Suggested Contextual Approach for IPV Research

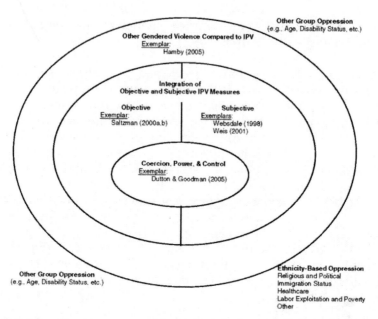

Note: Information at every contextual level informs all others in an iterative and embedded fashion. Top Level consists of cultural oppression of all types represented by text outside the circles that is coupled with the first outer circle where IPV is compared to other gendered violence. Middle Level is represented by the next layered circle where both objective and subjective IPV measures are obtained and integrated. Individual Level is represented at the inner-most circle through examination of ongoing coercion, power, and control within intimate relationships. Exemplars of such research are provided at each level (see text for more explanation).

RE-EMBEDDING IPV
WITHIN THE GENERAL SOCIAL CONTEXT

The Widespread Oppression of Women

As Chesney-Lind and Pasko (2004) have noted, being female within our culture comes at a price. In terms of sexual or physical victimization and exploitation, as well as a relative lack of economic earning power, being female is a distinct and well documented drawback. While it is known that women are blocked on many other fronts from enjoying control over their own bodies or other basic human rights (e.g., Watts & Zimmerman, 2002; see Figure 1), due to space constraints the section below will focus only on violent victimization, racism, and economic disparities as examples. While one would think that this overarching social context would be well understood and thus reflected in current scholarly academic discourse about women's use of IPV, largely it is not and has yet to be rectified. To this disappointing yet necessary end, a short review is presented below as a reminder of the violent, racial, and economic oppression women still face today, and as a model with which we may begin to re-embed the issue of women's use of IPV.

Information About Gender, Race, and Violence

Lethal violence. While it is clear that, overall, males are overwhelmingly both the victims and perpetrators of homicide (Craven, 1997; Federal Bureau of Investigation, 2002), IPV-related homicides are a different matter. Paulozzi, Saltzman, Thompson, and Holmgren (2001) examined IPV-related homicide data collected between 1981 and 1998 and found that rates had declined 47.2%, and that the decline was due to a much larger reduction for male homicide victims (67.8%) over this time period while females still had a roughly similar risk. Fox and Zawitz (2003) have shown that this overall downward trend in IPV-related homicides has continued in the few years since 1998. However, a striking finding remains: while the number of IPV-related homicide victims in the year 1976 were roughly equal for males (1,357) and females (1,600), in 2000 the number of male victims had declined drastically (440) compared to the number of female victims (1,247; Fox & Zawitz). Thus, while IPV-related homicides have declined overall, that decline is mainly due to the reduction in males being killed by their partners, while women are still dying in close to the same numbers as 30 years ago.

In terms of race and ethnicity, Fox and Zawitz (2003) found that Blacks were 6 times more likely to be victims of any type of homicide and 7 times more likely to commit murder when compared to Whites, an over-representation that has changed little over time. However, similarly to the overall decline in all types of homicides shown above, IPV-related homicides declined from 1976 to 2000 for all racial groups, with the exception of the number of White females killed (Fox & Zawitz).

The most important point here is that the vast majority of individuals committing homicide are male, regardless of age or ethnicity. In short, homicide perpetrators are men. The vast majority of intimates killed by a partner are women, and the perpetrators are male. In addition, people of color are disproportionately both victims and perpetrators of general homicide in relation to their actual numbers in the population. Furthermore, reductions in IPV homicide rates (both victimization and perpetration) have been seen for every segment in the population during the last few years, with the exception of White female IPV homicide victims.

Non-lethal sexual/physical violence. Recently, the American Psychological Association (APA; 2007) released the *Report on the APA Task Force on the Sexualization of Girls*. The Task Force synthesized available research evidence that shows the high level of sexualization girls and young women are subjected to within contemporary North American culture. The report showed how such gender-discriminatory sexualization occurs when:

> ... a person's value comes only from ... sexual appeal or behavior to the exclusion of other characteristics; a person is held to a standard that equates physical attractiveness ... with being sexy; a person is sexually objectified - that is, made into a thing for other's sexual use ... [and] sexuality is inappropriately imposed upon a person. (p. 2)

As Gavey (2005) has noted, such imposed sexuality is so common for females in Western culture that it has become almost invisible. Because sexualization is almost always related to females and not males, we forget such cultural influences at our own peril when investigating IPV.

Indeed, while girls and boys are victimized at roughly the same aggregate rates for simple and aggravated physical assaults, as girls progress to the age of 18, the risk of sexual and physical assault *combined* increases until it surpasses that of boys (Finkelhor & Asdigian, 1996; Finkelhor, Ormon, Turner, & Hamby, 2005). For example, Snyder and colleagues (Snyder, 2000; Snyder & Sickmund, 1999) found that 86% of all sexual assaults were perpetrated against females regardless of victim age, and that the proportion of female victims increased with age until it reached over 95% for all age groups 18 or above. Furthermore, it was found that males are the primary perpetrators of sexual assault and constituted the vast majority of all offenders, regardless of the age of the victim (Snyder; Snyder & Sickmund; U.S. Department of Justice, 2000). Rape statistics also show that adult women are 13 to 23 times more likely than men to be raped or sexually assaulted by intimates, acquaintances, or strangers (Craven, 1997). In 1999, women reported 91,740 rapes or sexual assaults at the hands of an intimate, with the incident rates peaking between the ages of 16 and 34 (Rennisen, 2002). It should not be surprising, then, that women are predominantly the victims of IPV when both sexual and physical assaults are combined (Malloy, McCloskey, Grigsby, & Gardner, 2003).

Similar to the rape statistics above, 62% of all non-lethal physical victimizations of females were perpetrated by known intimates, family members, friends, or acquaintances. Conversely, 64% of male physical assault victimizations were perpetrated by strangers. Regardless of whether the victim was a female or male, perpetrators of non-lethal physical violence were overwhelmingly male (Craven, 1997; Rennison & Rand, 2003). Furthermore, compared to men, women are overwhelmingly victimized within the home (Craven, 1997; Rennison, 2003; Rennison & Welchans, 2000). Thus, the majority of physically and sexually violent behavior against women is committed by known others (intimates, friends, family members, and acquaintances), and males are overwhelmingly the perpetrators of these crimes.

Concerning violence and ethnicity, Rennison and Rand (2003) reported declines in overall non-lethal violent victimization for all races between 1993 and 2002 in the U.S. Because Whites presently constitute the majority of the population, it should not be surprising that they constitute the single largest group of violent victims and perpetrators overall (Hobbs & Stoops, 2002; Simon, Mercy, & Perkins, 2001). However, when victimization and perpetration are expressed as percentages of the general population by ethnic distribution, another map emerges. People of color are both victims and perpetrators of non-lethal violence at higher rates per capita than Whites.

In summary, results for non-lethal sexual/physical violence are similar to those found for homicides: men are physically and sexually violent. When sexual assaults are combined with physical assaults, females of all ages are victimized at much higher rates than males. Finally, when adjusted for population, people of color are at much higher risk for overall non-lethal victimization and perpetration compared to their White counterparts.

Information About Gender, Race, and Economic Oppression

Poverty by gender and race. Data from the National Center for Children in Poverty (NCCP), housed at Columbia University, paint a harsh economic picture (Bennett & Lu, 2000; Gershoff, 2003; Lu & Koball, 2003; Song & Lu, 2002). Researchers from the NCCP suggest that

while the federal definition of poverty is currently $18,400 for a family
of four (Gershoff; Lu & Koball), a more accurate cut-off would be
roughly double that level (approximately $37,000 annually). By using
the NCCP's more accurate cut-off levels, derived by taking into consideration the steadily rising costs of food, housing, transportation, and
child care, nearly 40% of children in the U.S. live in poverty (Lu &
Koball). While the single largest category of low-income children are
White (10.9 million), they represent only 25% of all White children in
contrast to 62% of all Latino children and 58% of all Black children
(NCCP, 2004). In addition, children of single mothers are about five
times more likely to live in poverty than children living with two parents
(Song & Lu), and yet 84% of all poor children have at least one employed parent (NCCP). This counterintuitive result reflects gender
disparities in income between adult men and women (see below).

    While in some cases poor male children and adolescents are able to
escape poverty on their own during adulthood, the chances of a young
female lifting herself out of poverty without the "help of a man" are
much less. Unfortunately, poverty in the U.S. is a widespread and
gendered phenomenon. If we use only the official government estimate
of 35 million people living in poverty, we will still see a disparity between the genders: overall, more women live in poverty than do men
(Cancian & Meyer, 2000). In addition, the large pay gap between men
and women persists across the lifespan even today (Cancian & Meyer;
DeNavas-Walt, Cleveland, & Webster, 2002; Rose & Hartmann, 2004).

    Racial disparities also show distinct patterns in the way poverty is
dispersed. Bishaw and Iceland (2003) report that while 12.4% of the entire U.S. population currently lives in poverty, only 9.1% of Whites and
12.6% of Asians live below the poverty line. Compare this to approximately 25% of African-Americans and Native-Americans living in
poverty, or 24% of Hispanics living in poverty (Bishaw & Iceland).

    Wage gaps by gender and race. While results from the most recent
U.S. Census Bureau data suggest that, overall, women earn about 77
cents for every male dollar earned (DeNavas-Walt et al., 2002; Weinberg, 2003), it was found that earning power varied by race. Asian females make about 75 cents of every dollar earned by a White male,
followed by White females (70 cents), African-American females (62.5
cents), Native-American females (57.8 cents), and Hispanic females
(52.5 cents; Caiazza, Shaw, & Werschkul, 2004). It should not be surprising then that women of color per capita are much more likely to live
in poverty than White women, or that obvious variations in male wage
earnings based on ethnicity are evident (Caiazza et al., 2004). Overall,

White males are the largest wage earners, followed by males of color, White females, and females of color. Researchers from the Institute of Women's Policy Research in Washington, DC have shown that when a male and female cohort within the U.S. were followed for an entire 15 year period (instead of measures taken at one point in time by the Census Bureau), women workers in their prime made only 38% of what prime-age males earned (Rose & Hartmann, 2004). These researchers also found that, of those adults who worked every year and made less than $15,000 annually, over 90% were female. Thus, there are major effects on earning power due to gender segregation (i.e., traditionally male and female job types), and without connection to men, women are not insulated from low income levels due to gender-related job segregation and wage gaps (Rose & Hartmann).

Agars (2004) provided a compelling model of the cumulative effects of discrimination against women in the workplace. Initial small discriminatory "effect sizes" (e.g., being passed over for a promotion or raise, or being hired at lower pay than a male with similar background/credentials) translated into a huge negative impact on women's income over the long-term, regardless of the number of "breaks" taken from employment outside the home by either gender (Rose & Hartmann, 2004). Cumulative effects of small discriminatory job practices seem to start a statistical "snow-ball" effect from which women simply cannot recover (Agars; Rose & Hartmann; Lips, 2003; Negrey, Golin, Lee, Mead, & Gault, 2001). Even when women enter into male jobs, they are still paid less than men for equal work. An especially telling result from Rose and Hartmann's analysis was that when men entered jobs thought of as traditionally female, males still made more then their female counterparts.

Besides the observable gender-based discrepancies in earning power that still exist in the U.S., there are other economic barriers that keep women in poverty. Policies around childcare, welfare, and housing subsidies are specifically targeted against women and their children (Cancian & Meyer, 2000; Lovell & Emsellem, 2004; Negrey et al., 2001), and there are still huge gaps between men and women concerning pension/retirement coverage as evidenced by the overwhelming number of elderly women (but not men) in poverty (Hartmann & Lee, 2003; Shaw & Hill, 2001). Another major structural barrier against women's economic attainment is that work within the home does not have a dollar amount attached, with the exception of paid domestic help that only the well-off can afford (e.g., maids, nannies, butlers, etc.; Waring, 1988). Women rarely have the benefit of a stay-at-home wife to do the childcare and homemaking for free, let alone a paid nanny, maid, or butler, and many fathers who are absent do not provide childcare or pay child support (Rose & Hartmann, 2004; Waring). Precisely because women's unpaid responsibilities within the home so often center around childcare and home maintenance, it should not be surprising that without an adult male wage earner in the household, many children live in poverty along with their mothers (Rose & Hartmann). Thus, the evidence is overwhelming that women and children suffer from economic oppression within the U.S.

It seems evident from the review above that being female is a distinct disadvantage in our present culture. Women simply do not, as a group, have the social power of men. Women are harmed within our culture through physical and sexual violence as well as economic oppression that intersects with race and ethnicity, creating even further oppression for women of color. It is within this overarching social milieu that the issue of supposed IPV gender symmetry *must* be examined. The urgency and importance of this assertion is the exact reason why the review above was completed in such depth and length when compared to that given below.

IPV is an Exception to the Rule: The Importance of Comparing Gender-Related Violence Across Domains

Hamby (2005) provides an excellent exemplar for examining IPV within the context of other gender-related violent behavior found in our culture. Hamby reviewed the evidence that shows men are overwhelmingly the perpetrators across all types and categories of violent crime, from armed robbery to child abuse, when official records are examined (e.g., crime reports, emergency room visits, etc.). Thus, she suggests that the supposed gender symmetry found in self-report measures of IPV is an anomaly. Hamby states, "The proposition that men and women perpetrate partner violence equally would make partner violence unique in respect to other forms of interpersonal violence" (p. 725). She goes on to explain:

> As one of the co-authors of the CTS2 [a self-report measure of IPV], I am not suggesting that behavioral checklists have no place...it is an issue of sampling, rather often imprecisely, from different sets of behaviors. Behavioral self-report of partner vio-

lence shares much more, in terms of apparent gender parity and frequency, with other measures of relationship distress and conflict than it does with measures of crime. (p. 737)

Even so, women are being arrested for IPV in increasing numbers across the U.S. after the advent of changes in criminal justice system policy (O'Dell, this issue; Rajan & McCloskey, this issue), and some domestic violence researchers are more than happy to suggest that the actions of female primary perpetrators constitute a serious social problem that could well approach the seriousness of male violence (as evidence, see certain articles in the following recent publications addressing women's use of IPV: Bible, Dasgupta, & Osthoff, 2002-2003; Buttell & Carney, 2006; Cook & Swan, 2006; Frieze & McHugh, 2005; Hamberger, 2005; McHugh & Frieze, 2005). This type of stance could only be adopted if the overall pattern of gendered violent crime within our culture is ignored. Hamby (2005) suggests we adopt such a stance at our own peril. Instead, she asserts that viewing IPV within the context of other gender-related violence is crucial.

Is Objective Measurement Better than Subjective? The Importance of Using Both Approaches

The idea of using multiple types of measurement approaches to examine human phenomena is not new. It has been known for some time that the investigative methods we use will drive what we find (McHugh & Cosgrove, 2004; Wilbur, 1996, 2000). While Wilbur asserts that science has produced some of the most breathtaking technological advances ever seen and is associated with social change toward widespread democracy and an increase in the worth of the individual not previously seen in recorded history (see especially Wilbur [2000] for the arguments supporting these statements), nevertheless its objective methods have also been extremely over-used and over-applied to unsuited social domains, including IPV. Even though objective methods are rife with problems due to such things as underreporting and response biases of all kinds, Saltzman (2002a,b) provides a summarization of the best known objective approaches to IPV measurement as exemplars to follow.

Wilbur (1996, 2000) asserted that actual human knowledge is not limited to only external, measurable actions, and that subjective types of knowing are just as valuable but rarely tapped because they require a *dialogue* to investigate. In other words, someone has to *talk to the individual, or immerse themselves in the culture,* to understand subjective human knowledge. Once this happens, understanding becomes a "shared subjective" where objectification fades then disappears. This of course is anathema to the objective scientific method. However, unbelievably rich and depthful information is obtained when we use such approaches, as exemplified by Websdale's (1998) ethnographic study with rural battered women or Weis' (2001) narrative analyses of battered women's stories.

A full accounting of IPV must include extensive information from both objective and subjective domains, leaving neither out. As this information is gathered, a full-scale integration must take place. The two types of information must then be weighed, compared, and integrated, with ample room for the ability to state that IPV is multifaceted and multicausal. In other words, an either/or mentality creates a shut-down within integration efforts, and only a both/and approach will suffice. The field of domestic violence research is no different than other scientific specialties, and is top-heavy with questionable objective approaches while sorely lacking in subjective information of any type. This is noticeable in two ways: (a) the sheer volume of IPV information available based on objective sources compared to that based on subjective data, and (b) the presence of major inconsistencies (i.e., conflicting data concerning gender symmetry for IPV perpetration) within the objective approach that are inherently unresolvable from within that very approach. As the second step in recontextualizing IPV, elevating subjective measurements to equal research status and then integrating the results provide a more accurate and complete understanding. Without it, we lose a powerful research tool and remain in the dark about the true nature of IPV within our culture.

What Exactly is IPV? The Importance of Measuring Ongoing Coercion, Power, and Control at the Individual Level

It seems evident that most IPV measurement tools are objective in nature and also largely fail to capture ongoing coercion, power, and control patterns within intimate heterosexual relationships (e.g., Strauchler et al., 2004). Even though a critical examination of the weaknesses of our present measurement tools has been widely represented within the continuing controversy over supposed gender symmetry, few tools are available that capture coercion and control. Our ability to do so is especially crucial because IPV is unique in that, like only a handful of other criminal categories, victimization occurs within close interpersonal relationships over time.

Fortunately, Dutton and Goodman (2005) have recently provided a rich conceptualization of this phenomenon upon which our field can build. By operationalizing their IPV model of ongoing coercion and control, we can begin to reintroduce the real-world experiences of battered women to the equation. No longer do researchers need to respond to assertions that "all slaps are created equal," and we can instead turn our time and resources to creating both objective and subjective measures of coercion, getting at the very heart of IPV.

SUMMARY

For our field to truly understand women's use of IPV, it is crucial that the following three steps be taken by researchers to put context back into the equation: (a) incorporate the effects of multiple oppressions women face within the context of predominantly male offending across different types of violent criminal categories (top level); (b) integrate findings from both objective and subjective research methods that will require elevating subjective approaches to the same status as objective (middle level); and (c) centralize the issue of ongoing patterns of coercion, power, and control within our definitions of IPV (individual level).

CONCLUSIONS

In the words of Bloom and Reichert (1998):

Sexism produces an unhealthy imbalance of power between the genders, which is maintained by violence or the threat of violence and is strongly reinforced by male conditioning to violence. Economic inequality breeds extremes of poverty and racism that serve to justify the scapegoating of people of color, situations that are breeding grounds for violence...the combined effect of all these factors is to create a sense of existential confusion, a profound questioning of purpose and meaning that so characterizes the social environment of the late twentieth century. (p. 4)

I would add that this confusion extends into the present. The discourse within the field of domestic violence research is currently polarized between those who cannot or will not take into account women's overall cultural oppression when they examine women's use of IPV, and those who insist upon it. Currently, those who will not take such contextualization into account assert that women are as likely to be IPV primary perpetrators as men within the population, and that women's IPV is a serious public health problem in need of concentrated attention and intervention. In addition, when their methods are criticized, researchers in this camp may accuse their critics of stridently enforcing political correctness or even hiding evidence that women are primary perpetrators on a large scale.

Those who insist on including cultural oppression in their analyses recognize that of course women can be primary perpetrators, but that the problem rests in the sheer number of male-perpetrated IPV that is elevated in seriousness to the level of a crime. In addition, when their methods are criticized, researchers in this camp may accuse their critics of creating gender symmetry where there is none or even fabricating evidence through wrong-headed methodology. Individuals on both sides of the fence accuse the other of intolerance and blindly furthering their own political agendas. Currently, those sitting on the fence are seemingly being torn off (or torn in half). Obviously, I am solidly in the latter camp. Nevertheless, the present effort is offered in the spirit of bringing our field out of this morass and into a more comprehensive and culturally informed approach.

REFERENCES

Agars, M. D. (2004). Reconsidering the impact of gender stereotypes on the advancement of women in organizations. *Psychology of Women Quarterly, 28,* 103-111.

American Psychological Association. (2007). *Report of the APA Task Force on the sexualization of girls.* Washington, DC: Author.

Anderson, M. A., Gillig, P. M., Sitaker, M., McCloskey, K., Malloy, K., & Grigsby, N. (2003). "Why doesn't she just leave?": A descriptive study of victim reported impediments to her safety. *Journal of Family Violence, 18*(3), 151-155.

Bennett, N. G., & Lu, H.-H. (2000). *Child poverty in the States: Levels and trends from 1979 to 1998.* New York: National Center for Children in Poverty.

Bible, A., Dasgupta, S., & Osthoff, S. (Eds.). (2002-2003). Women's use of violence in intimate relationships: Part 1, 2, 3 [Special issues]. *Violence Against Women, 8*(11-12), 9(1).

Bishaw, A., & Iceland, J. (2003). *Poverty: 1999 - Census 2000 brief* (C2KBR-19). Washington, DC: U.S. Census Bureau.

Bloom, S. L., & Reichert, M. (1998). *Bearing witness: Violence and collective responsibility.* New York: Haworth.

Buttell, F. P., & Carney, M. M. (Eds.) (2006). *Women who perpetrate relationship violence: Moving beyond political correctness.* Binghamton, NY: Haworth Press.

Caiazza, A., Shaw, A., & Werschkul, M. (2004). *Women's economic status in the States: Wide disparities by race, ethnicity, and region* (5th Series). Washington, DC: Institute for Women's Policy Research.

Cancian, M., & Meyer, D. R. (2000). Work after welfare: Women's work effort, occupation, and economic well-being. *Social Work Research, 24,* 69-86.

Chesney-Lind, M., & Pasko, L. (2004). *The female offender: Girls, women, and crime* (2nd Ed.). Thousand Oaks, CA: Sage.

Cook, S., L., & Swan, S. C. (Eds.) (2006). Special issue. *Violence Against Women, 12*(11).

Craven, D. (1997). *Sex differences in violent victimization, 1994.* Washington, DC: U.S. Department of Justice Bureau of Justice Statistics [NCJ 164508].

DeNavas-Walt, C., Cleveland, R. W., & Webster, B. H. (2002). *Income in the United States: 2002.* Washington, DC: U.S. Census Bureau, Current Population Reports [P60-221].

Dutton, M. A., & Goodman, L. A. (2005). Coercion in intimate partner violence: Toward a new conceptualization. *Sex Roles, 52*(11-12), 743-757.

Eisler, R. (1987). *The chalice and the blade: Our history, our future.* New York: HarperCollins.

Faludi, S. (1991). *Backlash: The undeclared war against women.* New York: Crown.

Federal Bureau of Investigation. (2002). *Crime in the United States, Uniform Crime Reports, 2002.* Washington, DC: U.S. Department of Justice.

Finkelhor, D., & Asdigian, N. L. (1996). Risk factors for youth victimization: Beyond a lifestyles/routine activities theory approach. *Violence and Victims, 11*(1), 3-19.

Finkelhor, D., Ormrod, R., Turner, H., & Hamby, S. L. (2005). The victimization of children and youth: A comprehensive national survey. *Child Maltreatment, 10*(1), 5-25.

Fox, J. A., & Zawitz, M. W. (2003). *Homicide trends in the United States: 2000 update.* Washington, DC: U.S. Department of Justice, Bureau of Justice Statistics Crime Data Brief [NCJ-197471].

Frieze, I. H., & McHugh, M. C. (Eds.) (2005). Special issue: Female violence against intimate partners. *Psychology of Women Quarterly, 29*(3).

Gavey, N. (2005). *Just sex? The cultural scaffolding of rape.* New York: Routledge.

Gershoff, E. (2003, September). *Low income and hardship among America's kindergartners.* New York: National Center for Children in Poverty.

Hamberger, L. K. (Ed.) (2005). Special issue on men's and women's use of intimate partner violence. *Violence and Victims, 20*(3).

Hamby, S. L. (2005). Measuring gender differences in partner violence: Implications from research on other forms of violence and socially undesirable behavior. *Sex Roles, 52*(11-12), 725-743.

Hartman, H., & Lee, S. (2003, April). *Social security: The largest source of income for both women and men in retirement.* Washington, DC: Institute for Women's Policy Research [IWPR-D455].

Hobbs, F., & Stoops, N. (2002). *Demographic trends in the 20th century: Census 2000 special reports* [CENSR-4]. Washington, DC: U.S. Government Printing Office, U.S. Census Bureau.

Johnson, M. P. (1995). Patriarchal terrorism and common couple violence: Two forms of violence against women. *Journal of Marriage and the Family, 57,* 283-294.

Lips, H. M. (2003). The gender pay gap: Concrete indicator of women's progress toward equality. *Analyses of Social Issues & Public Policy (ASAP), 3,* 87-109.

Lovell, V., & Emsellem, M. (2004). *Florida's unemployment insurance system: Barriers to program adequacy for women, low-wage and part-time workers, and workers of color.* Washington, DC: Institute for Women's Policy Research [IWPR-C354].

Lu, H.-H., & Koball, H. (2003, August). *The changing demographics of low-income families and their children.* New York: National Center for Children in Poverty.

Malloy, K. A., McCloskey, K. A., Grigsby, N., & Gardner, D. (2003). Women's use of violence within intimate relationships. *Journal of Aggression, Maltreatment, and Trauma, 6,* 37-59.

McHugh, M. C., & Cosgrove, L. (2004). Feminist research methods: Studying women and gender. In M. A. Paludi (Ed.), *Praeger guide to the psychology of gender* (pp. 155-182). Westport, CT: Praeger.

McHugh, M. C., & Frieze, I. H. (Eds.) (2005). Special issue: Understanding gender and intimate partner violence: Theoretical and empirical approaches. *Sex Roles, 52*(11-12).

National Center for Children in Poverty. (2004, May). *Low-income children in the United States.* New York: Author. Retrieved June 17, 2006 http://www.nccp.org

Negrey, C., Golin, S., Lee, S., Mead, H., & Gault, B. (2001). *Working first but working poor: The need for education and training following welfare reform, executive summary.* Washington, DC: Institute for Women's Policy Research [IWPR-D443].

O'Dell, A. (2007). Why do police arrest victims of domestic violence? The need for comprehensive training and investigative protocols. *Journal of Aggression, Maltreatment, & Trauma, 15*(3/4), 53-73.

Paulozzi, L. J., Saltzman, L. E., Thompson, M. P., & Holmgren, P. (2001). Surveillance for homicide among intimate partners: United States 1981-1998. *Morbidity and Mortality Weekly Report, 50*(SS03), 1-16.

Rajan, M., & McCloskey, K. A. (2007). Victims of intimate partner violence: Arrest rates across recent studies. *Journal of Aggression, Maltreatment, & Trauma, 15*(3/4), 27-52.

Rennison, C. M. (2002). *Rape and sexual assault: Reporting to police and medical attention, 1992-2000.* Washington, DC: U.S. Department of Justice, Bureau of Justice Statistics Selected Findings [NCJ-194530].

Rennison, C. M. (2003). *Intimate partner violence, 1993-2001.* Washington, DC: U.S. Department of Justice, Bureau of Justice Statistics Crime Data Brief [NCJ-197838].

Rennison, C. M., & Rand, M. R. (2003). *Criminal victimization, 2002.* Washington, DC: U.S. Department of Justice, Office of Justice Programs [NCJ-199994].

Rennison, C. M., & Welchans, S. (2000). *Intimate partner violence.* Washington, DC: U.S. Department of Justice, Bureau of Justice Statistics Special Report [NCJ-178247].

Rose, S. J., & Hartmann, H. I. (2004). *Still a man's labor market: The long-term earnings gap.* Washington, DC: Institute for Women's Policy Research [IWPR-C355].

Saltzman, L. E. (2000a). Building data systems for monitoring and responding to violence against women, part I. *Violence Against Women, 6*(7).

Saltzman, L. E. (2000b). Building data systems for monitoring and responding to violence against women, part II. *Violence Against Women, 6*(8).

Shaw, L., & Hill, C. (2001, April). *The gender gap in pension coverage: Women working full-time are catching up, but part-time workers have been left behind.* Washington, DC: Institute for Women's Policy Research [IWPR-E506].

Simon, T., Mercy, J., & Perkins, C. (2001). *Injuries from violent crime, 1992-1998* [NCJ-168633]. Washington, DC: U.S. Department of Justice and U.S. Department of Health and Human Services.

Snyder, H. N. (2000). *Sexual assault of young children as reported to law enforcement: Victim, offender, and incident characteristics* (NCJ 182990). Washington, DC: U.S. Department of Justice, Bureau of Justice Statistics (www.ncjrs.org).

Snyder, H. N., & Sickmund, M. (1999). *Juvenile offenders and victims: 1999 National Report* (NCJ 178257). Washington, DC: U.S. Department of Justice, Office of Juvenile Justice and Delinquency Prevention (www.ncjrs.org).

Song, Y., & Lu, H.-H. (2002, March). *Early childhood and poverty: A statistical profile.* New York: National Center for Children in Poverty.

Strauchler, R., McCloskey, K., Malloy, K., Sitaker, M., Grigsby, N., & Gillig, P. (2004). Humiliation, manipulation, and control: Evidence of centrality in domestic violence against an adult partner. *Journal of Family Violence, 19*(6), 339-354.

Straus, M. A. (2006). Future research on gender symmetry in physical assaults on partners. *Violence Against Women, 12*(11), 1089-1097.

U.S. Department of Justice. (2000). *Children as victims: 1999 National Report Series Juvenile Justice Bulletin* (NCJ 180753). Rockville, MD: Juvenile Justice Clearinghouse. Retrieved June 2, 2004 from http://www.ncjrs.org

Waring, M. (1988). *If women counted: A new feminist economics.* San Francisco, CA: Harper & Row.

Watts, C., & Zimmerman, C. (2002). Violence against women: Global scope and magnitude. *Lancet, 359*(9313), 1232-1237.

Websdale, N. (1998). *Rural women battering and the justice system: An ethnography.* Thousand Oaks, CA: Sage.

Weinberg, D. H. (2003, September). *Press briefing on 2002 income and poverty estimates.* Washington, DC: U.S. Census Bureau. Retrieved June 18, 2006, http://www.census.gov/hhes/income/income02/prs03asc.html

Weis, L. (2001). Race, gender, and critique: African-American women, White women, and domestic violence in the 1980s and 1990s. *Signs: Journal of Women in Culture & Society, 27*, 139-169.

Wilbur, K. (1996). *A brief history of everything.* Boston, MA: Shambhala.

Wilbur, K. (2000). *Sex, ecology, spirituality: The spirit of evolution* (2nd ed.). Boston, MA: Shambhala.

Submitted: April 9, 2007
Revised: May 30, 2007
Accepted: May 30, 2007

Victims of Intimate Partner Violence: Arrest Rates Across Recent Studies

Mekha Rajan
Kathy A. McCloskey

A SHORT HISTORY OF INTIMATE PARTNER VIOLENCE AS A SOCIO-LEGAL PROBLEM IN THE U.S.

Changes for the Better: Socio-Legal Policies Concerning IPV

In the U.S., social changes have prompted federal and state govern-ments to take a stronger stance in curbing intimate partner violence (IPV) over the last 40 years. Throughout history, however, this was not always the case. Instead, Western cultures have often condoned those conditions in which wives had to endure the legal, physical, and mental rule of husbands (Bachman & Coker, 1995; Hirschel, Hutchison, Dean, & Mills, 1992). Indeed, violence against women has been implicitly condoned throughout U.S. history (Mills, 1999). Fortunately, as time progressed and reform efforts in the early 1900s were successful (e.g., suffrage), women's and victims' rights proponents began to gain both voice and ground. However, it was not until the civil rights movement of the 1960s that concrete changes arose.

During this time, advocates for battered women began speaking out against IPV and calling for greater batterer accountability as well as safe outlets for victims (Bennett, Goodman, & Dutton, 1999; Dasgupta, 2003; Fagan, 1996). Changes as a consequence of advocacy helped raise awareness of IPV as human rights and public health issues, with the rates and patterns of violence in U.S. homes taking center stage (Bachman & Coker, 1995). As a result, battered women's shelters, rape crisis centers, and hotlines were soon opened, allowing victims safe alternatives as an escape from the violence (Carlson & Nidey, 1995; Kim, 2004).

Nevertheless, a large majority of law enforcement agencies in the U.S. continued using a 'hands-off' IPV policy prior to the precedent-setting legal reforms of the 1970s (Fagan, 1996). Often, police officers responding to IPV scenes did not view IPV as appropriate police business, while paradoxically many law enforcement officials believed that IPV situations were dangerous and could lead to officer harm or fatality (Fagan). As a result, law enforcement officials were often left to mediate IPV situations or use crisis intervention techniques as part of a less active approach (Bohmer, Brandt, Bronson, & Hartnett, 2002; Bourg & Stock, 1994; Fagan). In practice, this meant that officers usually required batterers to simply leave the situation for a "cooling off" period before returning home, resulting in few negative consequences as a result of their violent behavior and little safety for their victims (Maxwell, Garner, & Fagan, 2002). Not surprisingly, these law enforcement practices often failed to curb the violence.

It also became increasingly apparent that law enforcement officers often treated IPV as lesser crimes than those assaults involving strangers (Carlson & Nidey, 1995; Feder, 1998). Additionally, both advocates and law enforcement officials began to realize that previously used intervention techniques, such as mediation at the scene, were not effective in preventing further violence (Maxwell et al., 2002). Instead, proponents sought to criminalize IPV and ensure a strong response from law enforcement in hopes of deterring batterers and holding them responsible for their actions (Fagan, 1996; Dasgupta, 2003). One result of such efforts included the actions of the Law Enforcement Assistantship Administration. This administration passed reforms that included the promotion of mandatory arrest laws and intervention programs for women who attempted to seek recourse against their batterers, promoting an improved IPV response from federal and state organizations (Fagan).

Prior to such legal reforms, women faced many difficulties in bringing charges against their batterers or obtaining and enforcing protective court orders. State and federal reforms, however, allowed victims of IPV to access emergency relief, regardless if they were divorced, separated, or cohabitating with their batterers. An example of such a reform was the passage of the Pennsylvania Protection from Abuse Act of 1976, which allowed relief in the means of protective orders to all IPV victims within that state (Pennsylvania Supreme Court Committee on Racial and Gender Bias, 2003). Thus, the 1970s ended with reforms that offered many victims new protections from their abusers and opened the door for further research and policy change.

In the 1980s, victims were offered even greater legal protection as a result of one particular research experiment as well as a series of lawsuits. In 1981, a large scale study was conducted by the Minneapolis Police Department to assess the extent to which arrest prevented further abuse in IPV cases (Bachman & Coker, 1995). The authors of the study, Sherman and Berk, assigned officers to one of three intervention strategies in response to IPV. The officer arrested the offender in the first intervention. For the second intervention, the officer had the batterer leave the premises for 24 hours and return later. In the third intervention, the officer was expected only to restore order at the scene. The results of the study showed that arrest had the greatest impact in preventing future violence (Berk, Campbell, Klap, & Western, 1992). Findings from this experiment became widely known and were instrumental in changing the public's traditional viewpoint concerning IPV. It became common knowledge that IPV is a legal matter that should result in formal repercussions and sanctions for the batterer (Fagan, 1996). The study also fostered further interest and subsequent research into the efficacy of police response to IPV situations, spawning more debate and legal change (see below).

During this same time frame, victims of IPV began filing lawsuits against certain jurisdictions as retribution for damages due to failure to provide citizen protection through appropriate justice system intervention (Bohmer et al., 2002). In the civil case of *Bruno v. Codd* (1978), a group of battered wives filed suit against the New York City Police Department (NYPD), probation officers, and clerks of the family court for failing to protect them from their abusive husbands. The survivors accused the NYPD of discriminatory and abusive treatment in neglecting to arrest their batterers and failing to enforce protective orders. In a similar case, *Thurman v. City of Torrington* (1984), the plaintiff sued the City of Torrington, CT and its police department for lack of action in protecting female citizens from assaults by their male partners. The case dealt with a victim who had contacted the Torrington Police Department about the multiple threats made against her and her son by her estranged husband. The plaintiff's husband had also violated a two year court order of protection. These claims, the plaintiff argued, were ignored or dismissed. The situation escalated so severely and the police responded so poorly that the estranged husband kicked and stabbed the plaintiff in the yard of her house in plain view of police officers who stood by as passive witnesses. Needless to say, the court ruled for the plaintiff and not only upheld the duty of civic officials to protect all citizens from harm, but also found that the victim's rights under the 14th amendment were violated. The court also affirmed that the plaintiff was a victim of discriminatory classification because less protection was offered to an IPV victim than would have been offered during another type of assault. The cases outlined above resulted in successful court victories and gains for victims.

Pressure on state and local governments resulting from such lawsuits, concomitant with widespread dissemination of the results from the Minneapolis Domestic Violence Experiment, eventually led to widespread changes in arrest policies (Bachman & Coker, 1995; Fagan, 1996). The new policies, for example, required law enforcement officials to arrest offenders who had violated protective orders (Dugan, 2003). Throughout the 1980s, state and local legislatures across the U.S. began passing laws that criminalized violence in domestic situations, and police were mandated to practice more stringent arrest policies regardless of whether or not officers had warrants or had actually witnessed the assaults (Carlson & Nidey, 1995; Maxwell et al., 2002). By 1989, all 50 states and the District of Columbia had provisions for civil protective orders, providing victims relief and safety from their abusers (Goodmark, 2004). Thus, the 1980s ended with nationwide reforms in arrest laws and protective orders that recognized the rights of IPV victims and the need to keep them safe (Fagan).

The 1990s signified even greater changes in the criminal justice system, especially those aimed at increasing aid to victims as well as legal sanctions against batterers (Fagan, 1996). In 1994, the federal government passed the Violence Against Women Act (VAWA) (Dasgupta, 2003; Library of Congress, 1994), and shortly thereafter, the Family Protection and Domestic Violence Intervention Act was passed, creating a standardized protocol for responding to IPV offenders at the scene (State of New York, 1998). This latter Act redefined family violence as that which occurs against any member of the same family or household instead of only between legally married heterosexual couples, and also called for the arrest of batterers as the preferred intervention by law enforcement (Haviland, Frye, Rajah, Thukral, & Trinity, 2001). In an effort to insure that thorough investigations were conducted at the scene, this reform also required officers to make a written report whether or not an arrest was made and to include more extensive documentation of the incident, such as victim and witness statements (e.g., *Groves v. State University of New York*, 2000).

In those U.S. jurisdictions that passed mandatory arrest laws or otherwise adopted such policies, officers were required to make an arrest if they had probable cause to believe that violence had taken place (Goodmark, 2004; Mills, 1999). With the advent of mandatory arrest across many jurisdictions, more cases were being sent to the courts, prompting states to pass even more stringent laws regarding the prosecution of offenders with the adoption of mandatory sentencing and no-drop policies (Bennett et al., 1999; Carlson & Nidey, 1995; Goodmark). Some states required offenders to be sent to jail for a period of time and/or attend batterer treatment programs (Carolson & Nidey). In addition, no-drop policies prevented victims from dropping charges against their offenders due to fear of batterer retaliation. Regardless if victims wished to drop the charges or refused to cooperate, prosecutors could continue to pursue legal action against abusers by using victims' statements at the time of arrest in addition to police evidence and testimony (Bennett et al.; Mills, 1998, 1999). Thus, no-drop and mandatory arrest policies reduced or removed the ability of the victim to influence the decision to arrest or prosecute the batterer, which paved the way for heated debate and controversy. For instance, victims and battered women's advocates were understandably outraged that victims were being prosecuted in some jurisdictions for failing to testify against their batterers (Goodmark).

As the decades passed, one message became clear. Overall, the U.S. was taking a more strict and active role in curbing IPV. No longer was IPV considered a private matter, but instead a legal and social concern for all citizens. Subsequent legal and social reforms offered victims greater options and protections in an attempt to deter further violence by holding batterers accountable. The increase in victim services also helped battered women escape the violence and seek reparations. Despite these positive gains, victims faced other hurdles in contending with the unintended consequences of policy changes. The more stringent policies favored active measures in IPV cases and led to an increase in the number of victims prosecuted or otherwise pressured for failure to testify (Bohmer et al., 2002). Even more disturbingly, victims were increasingly being arrested at the IPV scene (see below). The rise in victim arrest rates was attributed to not only poor implementation at the scene and the lack of proper enforcement of new policies, but also the inevitable social backlash where women are now often considered equal to men as primary IPV perpetrators.

Two Steps Forward and One Step Back: Backlash Concerning Gender Symmetry

The increase in victim arrest rates followed a change in perception from a primarily male abuser/female victim dyad to supposed gender symmetry (Henning & Renauer, 2005; Henning, Renauer, & Holdford, 2006). The first such documented backlash can be traced to the late 1970's as a result of Straus and colleagues' original studies using the Conflict Tactic Scale (CTS). Straus and colleagues first provided research support for symmetry in men and women's IPV perpetration based on self-reports using the CTS (e.g., Steinmetz & Straus, 1974; Straus & Gelles, 1986), and these findings were used to promote the concept of the 'battered husband syndrome' (Anderson, 2005). As a result, victims were being labeled as primary batterers and considered as violent as their male counterparts (e.g., Renzetti, 1996). While this viewpoint lost favor in the 1980s and the early part of the 1990s due to well-known problems with CTS methodology (e.g., poor convergent/divergent construct validity due to a non-contextual approach), this viewpoint is once again making a comeback as a legitimate stance (Straus, 2006; for recent critiques of this stance, see Hamberger, 2005a; Hamby, 2005; Malloy, McCloskey, Grigsby, & Gardner, 2003).

Support for the idea that we are currently in the middle of another large change in social perception can be found in preliminary reports from Straus' (2004, 2005) International Dating Violence Study (IDVS). Straus once again found that, using the CTS, young adult women and men report roughly equal amounts of violent acts against their dating partners. Regardless of the country in which the respondents reside, this pattern of results held. These results further demonstrate the lack of construct validity within Strauss' approach, especially since it has been well known for years that particular countries exist along a continuum concerning human rights abuses against women (i.e., severe status inequalities found in places such as fundamentalist Islamic nations, African locations, or Pacific Rim countries versus less status inequalities in some Westernized countries; World Health Organization, 2005). Yet another phenomenon in support of the present change within the IPV gender zeitgeist has been the recent increase in scholarly special issue journal publications focusing exclusively on women as primary IPV perpetrators (Bible, Dasgupta, & Osthoff, 2002-2003; Buttell & Carney, 2006; Cook & Swan, 2006; Frieze & McHugh, 2005; Hamberger, 2005b; McHugh & Frieze, 2005).

While some women are primary IPV perpetrators, as a public health issue the phenomenon pales considerably when compared to the overwhelming social costs of widespread violent male behavior of which IPV is just one part. Not surprisingly, the increased attention on women has been used quite effectively by those who wish to convince others that women are as violent as men within intimate relationships. Disturbingly, advocates for the men's rights movement cite just these types of research studies because they support the viewpoint that women are as likely as men to be primary batterers (DeKeseredy, 1999). For example, one website cited results from studies using the CTS where the gender split was virtually equal (Middap, 2000, ¶ 9) as evidence that women are as violent as men. Certain sources dedicated to advancing the men's rights movement also state that in 15-38% of IPV cases the primary victim is male, but that these numbers are actually much higher because men are less likely to report being abused (*Men's Rights*, n.d., ¶ 11). Based on such reasoning, men's rights advocates conclude that the number of women should represent about 50% or more of all IPV cases in terms of arrest and prosecution, and they welcome the recent increase in women's arrests.

Perhaps one reason for the cyclical re-emergence of the belief that women are violent like men concerns the overall ineffectiveness of current public health approaches in reducing IPV. While it has been known for some time that IPV is but one type of overwhelmingly violent and oppressive male behavior found within our culture (including but not limited to general violent behavior against other men and children, homicide, sexual assault, economic exploitation, and the glorification of both male violence and female sexualization within the media; Boyle, 2005; Chesney-Lind & Pasko, 2004; Geffner, Sorenson, & Lundberg-Love, 1997), seldom do public health interventions approach the problem of male IPV as connected across these different domains (see Sitaker, this issue). An example of just such an ineffective public health approach in the U.S. is the focus on battered women's services within the last 40 years without a concomitant increase in widespread and coordinated interventions for curtailing the behavior of violent males. For instance, providing battered women with the increased means to escape their batterers correlates strongly with a steep reduction in the number of men killed by their intimate female partners, while there has been no such dramatic decrease in the number of women killed (e.g., Fox & Zawitz, 2006; Paulozzi, Saltzman, Thompson, & Holmgree, 2001). By focusing largely on helping battered women escape and/or increasing access to the legal system for protective orders, the actions of battered women were the primary target for intervention. This resulted in a very predictable outcome: men continued to murder their female partners in slightly reduced numbers, while their own risk of dying at the hands of their female intimate partners drastically decreased. Thus, this approach was effective, but with the wrong target population.

Yet another example concerns the inability to reproduce the original positive results from the Minnesota Police Department that had demonstrated that arrest and subsequent community control showed a definite reduction in future IPV perpetration by violent males. It seems that most, if not all, of the researchers at the replication sites could not secure the programmatic buy-in needed to standardize and therefore replicate police responses at the IPV scene, let alone ensure well-controlled and documented follow-up by probation/parole officers or otherwise create a coordinated community response (Buzawa & Buzawa, 2003; Mills, 1998, 1999). While a coordinated community response approach is most likely highly effective with male IPV perpetrators (with the exception of a few batterers fitting a particular profile), reproducing the positive Minnesota results has been virtually impossible due to a lack of multi-jurisdiction police department accountability and standardization (e.g., Buzawa & Buzawa; Klein, 2004; Mills). In other words, while everyone now seems to agree that an IPV victim can and should leave her batterer and society should provide the means across systems for her to do so, we are still largely hesitant to hold the batterer accountable for his actions, let alone provide systematic means to accomplish this. Such hesitancy fuels and sustains the opportunities for backlash.

The criminal justice system within the U.S. is not immune to such problems in social perception; indeed, the criminal justice system is embedded firmly within it. Those in charge of making primary batterer identifications, including police officers at the scene, prosecutors, and judges, are all potentially affected. It is not surprising, then, that this backlash can also be seen in the increased arrests of IPV victims. Because falsely arrested victims can be subject to potentially severe consequences, including negative legal, financial, employment, and child custody repercussions, we now turn to the recent increases in victim arrests and the factors that are associated with them.

VICTIM ARRESTS

The Numbers

Between 1991 and 2000, there was a 15.7% increase overall in the number of women arrested for all types of crimes, compared to a 3.9%

decrease in the overall arrest rates for men (Chesney-Lind, 2002). It is therefore not surprising that various authors have also noted a sobering and increasing trend in the number of IPV cases resulting in the erroneous arrest of the victim (see Table 1).

In 1991, the Family Violence Reporting Program, under the auspices of the Connecticut Department of Public Safety, conducted a

TABLE 1. Increased Arrest Rates of Battered Women since the Advent of Mandatory/Preferred Arrest Laws

Authors(s)	Increase?	
	Single Arrest	Dual Arrest
Bohmer et al. (2002)[a]	Yes	Yes
Chesney-Lind (2002)[a,b]	Yes	Yes
Family Violence Reporting Program (1991)[b]	--	Yes
Hamberger & Potente (1994)[a,b]	Yes	Yes
Haviland et al. (2001)[a,b]	Yes	Yes
Henning & Feder (2004)[a]	--	Yes
Klein (2004)[b,c]	Yes	Yes
Martin (1997)[a,b]	--	Yes
Miller (2001)[a]	Yes	--
Swan & Snow (2002)[b]	Yes	--

[a] Qualitative victim narratives and/or informal observation of author(s).
[b] Based on quantitative results from community data.
[c] Klein (2004) estimates that the overall increase in erroneous arrests of battered women now averages about 25-35% nationwide since the advent of mandatory/preferred arrest laws.
Note. Dashes indicate the arrest rate was not estimated or discussed.

study on the effects of mandatory arrest policy and found an increase in dual arrests with a 20.4% error on the officers' part in classifying victims as offenders. A 1999 report issued by the State of California also found that while IPV arrests across the state increased overall from 31,886 in 1988 to 56,892 in 1998, males dropped from 94% to 83.5% of all IPV arrests made within this time period, while females increased from 6% to 16.5% (State of California Office of the Attorney General, 1999). Thus, while IPV arrests of men proportionately decreased in California over a 10 year period, arrests of women increased almost three-fold. One reason associated with the overall rise in victim arrests is the poor implementation of pro-arrest and/or mandatory arrest statutes that were originally intended to ensure that batterers are held accountable across locations and jurisdictions (Chesney-Lind, 2002; Hamberger & Potente, 1994; Haviland et al., 2001; Henning & Feder, 2004; Klein, 2004; Martin, 1997; Miller, 2001; Swan & Snow, 2002).

Hamberger and Potente (1994) reported that after mandatory and preferred arrest policies went into affect, there was a twelve-fold increase in the number of women arrested within one particular geographical location, while arrest rates for men increased only two-fold. Although legislatures have attempted to create laws that are less confusing regarding the arrest of actual offenders at IPV scenes, dual arrest rates have nevertheless continued to increase over the years.

Between 1997 and 2001, Henning and Feder (2004) found that women were almost five times as likely to be involved in a dual arrest as men. In analyzing studies conducted across police jurisdictions, Haviland et al. (2001) found that after the enforcement of presumptive arrest policies, the average dual arrest rate of 4-12% rose considerably to 15-30%. While women made up about one fourth of these arrests (Haviland et al.), the authors concluded that due to failure by police departments to consistently report and collect data on dual arrests, it was difficult to get an accurate number of the victims actually dually arrested.

As further research was conducted to ascertain victim arrest rates, a profile of the 'arrested victim' emerged. Studies showed that victims were more likely to be dually arrested if they were cohabiting with their offenders, non-married, young (between the ages of 16 and 30), and involved in substance use (Finn, Blackwell, Stalans, Studdard, & Dugan, 2004; Martin, 1997). Other characteristics common among victims included suffering from depressive symptoms and being unemployed

(Dowd, Leisring, & Rosenbaum, 2005). Most importantly, however, dual arrest victims were much less likely to have engaged in previous violence than their perpetrators, and were likely to have been victims in prior incidents (Martin; Dowd et al.; Feder & Henning, 2005).

In response to the increase in dual arrests, the state of New York passed a Primary Physical Aggressor (PPA) provision (Haviland et al., 2001), which stated that in situations where there was reasonable cause to suspect both parties of violence, officers were required to evaluate four separate factors before an arrest can be made. The factors included ascertaining: (a) the extent of injuries for both parties, (b) whether one person had threatened future harm to the other, (c) which party had a previous history of violence, and (d) whether an individual was acting in self-defense. Although the law was passed to circumvent the shortcomings of previous presumptive policies, the statute had its own failures. Not only did it fail to protect victims against false accusations of violence by batterers, adherence to its principles of effectiveness and fairness was also lacking because it contained no enforcement or monitoring provisions. The results of Haviland et al.'s (2001) study evaluating arrest after the implementation of the PPA statute showed that the majority of dual arrest victims had civil protective orders previously violated by their abusers, had a prior history of victimization, and their offenders had a history of IPV. Thus, despite the PPA provision, over a third of dual arrests made clearly involved primary victims. The authors concluded that if the PPA provision was adequately followed, dual arrests would have been prevented in 60% of these cases (Haviland et al.).

A study conducted by Henning and Feder (2004) found that women were arrested in almost 17% of IPV incidents within the location they studied. However, Henning and Renauer (2005) found that as many as 62% of cases brought against women were later dropped or dismissed, or the women were found not guilty. This meant that only about 6-7% of the women arrested in their sample later pled or were found guilty of IPV. Furthermore, Swan and Snow (2002) reported that 34% of the women arrested in IPV cases were clearly classified as victims. Taken together, this suggests that one-half to three-quarters of female IPV arrests are erroneous. In addition, Table 2 shows that, on average across some of the recent studies in the U.S., only about 1-7% of all IPV arrests are of actual female primary perpetrators.

Possible Reasons for the Increase in Victim Arrests

Besides being quite disturbing, the results outlined above also raise an important question: Why are victims now being arrested in such high num-

TABLE 2. For Every IPV Arrest, How Many are Female Primary Perpetrators?[a]

Authors(s)	% Women Out of All IPV Arrests	% Women Arrested Are Actual Primary Perpetrators
Feder & Henning (2005)	16.3%[b]	--
Henning & Feder (2004)	17%[b]	--
Henning et al. (2006)	8-9%	1-5%[c]
Henning & Renauer (2005)	13.8%	6.6%[d]
O'Dell (this issue)	--	3%[e]
Swan & Snow (2002)	20%	2-5 %[c]

[a] Best-estimate averages from findings cited: One-half to three-quarters of all female IPV arrests are erroneous and only 1-7% of all IPV arrests are of actual female primary perpetrator.
[b] Samples may overlap among these two studies.
[c] Perpetrator status determined using classification scheme.
[d] Perpetrator status determined as those successfully prosecuted.
[e] Represents estimate from informal observations.
Note. Dashes indicate the arrest rate was not estimated. Adapted and updated from K. McCloskey, (2005, August), Battered Women Arrested for Domestic Violence . Paper presented at the meeting of the American Psychological Association, Washington, D.C.

bers? One answer lies with the cyclical cultural backlash zeitgeist currently found in the U.S., as reviewed above. Still other answers can be found in the manipulative behavior of batterers, the poor implementation of IPV statutes by police at the scene, and widely varying actions by prosecutors, judges, and probation/parole officers across jurisdictions.

Batterer manipulation of the criminal justice system. Thorough police investigations at the IPV scene are even more crucial when the manipulative behavior of the batterer is considered. When faced with the prospect of being arrested, charged, and prosecuted for IPV, batterers have learned to not only further control victims with fear and threats, but they have also learned to manipulate the legal system to their benefit (Bohmer et al., 2002; Haviland et al., 2001; Miller, 2001). Studies have shown that abusers have used "retaliatory arrests" by filing fabricated or embellished complaints against victims who have defended themselves (Haviland et al.). This is also prevalent in cases where batterers are threatened with losing custody of their children (Goodmark, 2004).

Furthermore, batterers can file for a civil protection order against their victims, even if the victim has already filed a complaint or obtained a protection order against the batterer (Goodmark). Thus, offenders are using the threat of legal action and possible arrest against their victims in order to maintain control. Unfortunately, batterers are learning how to use the criminal justice system to their advantage, potentially leading to the increase in victim arrests (Henning & Renauer, 2005; Miller).

Criminal justice system response. Police officers at the scene are vulnerable to batterer manipulation without training in IPV investigative procedures (O'Dell, this issue). Furthermore, police officers are more likely to arrest victims with particular characteristics, such as those who use alcohol or drugs, those with a prior history of being abused, and those who have no previous violent record (Belknap, 1995; Haviland et al., 2001). Women more susceptible to arrest are also those who do not fit the typical stereotype of 'the good victim' (Haviland et al.; Martin, 1997), such as women who are abrasive and argumentative, who are aggressive towards their abusers for any reason (including self-defense), or who otherwise fail to conform to traditional female gender roles (Robinson & Chandek, 2000; Saunders, 1995). It is not surprising, then, that studies have shown that an officer's own beliefs and attitudes about women and IPV can also impact the arrest decision (Finn et al., 2004; Martin). Finn et al. found that, in the absence of an adequate investigation, officers were more likely to view women as violent and men as faultless if the man exhibited visible injuries. The authors concluded that, overall, officers viewed women in a less positive manner. Indeed, victims who refuse to be passive participants within an abusive relationship often have a higher chance for arrest (Feder & Henning, 2005). Thus, officers' selective biases and stereotypes place victims at greater risk for arrest. This is true even though it has been known for some time that police training results in a decrease in erroneous IPV arrests (e.g., Mignon & Holmes, 1995).

In addition, a study conducted by Hartman and Belknap (2003) revealed that law enforcement officials viewed IPV cases and its victims as frustrating and not worthy of their time. Officers were also found to minimize the potential negative consequence of arrest for victims (Miller, 2001). Other law enforcement officials surveyed were reported as preferring the use of mediation at the scene, rather than arresting the offender (Belknap, 1995). In holding such beliefs, it is not hard to understand why so few officers take the time to properly investigate IPV situations and assess the primary perpetrator. Mandating officers to arrest, however, may not be the total solution. In fact, as Mills (1999) states, it is questionable as to whether depriving police of their own discretion in violent situations actually promotes efficacy and fairness within the community. Instead, as an unintended result, officers who harbor resentment towards IPV policies and its victims may become inefficient and perpetrate further injustice at the scene. Unfortunately, policy change without the concomitant social change can cause unintended consequences. In fact, this is a good recipe for creating and sustaining a backlash against victims in particular and women's rights in general.

These factors increase the chance that an erroneous victim arrest will be made. In such cases, officers may arrest both parties (Goodmark, 2004; O'Dell, this issue), thereby allowing officers to avoid liability and the responsibility of properly investigating the situation. In doing so, officers also ignore situations where victims have responded in self-defense (Bohmer et al., 2002; Mignon & Holmes, 1995), often because they are unwilling to evaluate IPV within the context of ongoing violence (Danis, 2003). Instead, law enforcement officials too often assess each case as a single event in time, ignoring the context of prior victimization, even when they have been called to a particular household in the past.

Across three counties within a particular state, Miller (2001) found that criminal justice and social service respondents agreed that the increase in victim arrests was a product of recent changes in public policy. Miller argued that this is a result of the lack of local resources to properly train officers with regard to the most effective police response at IPV scenes. Such hesitance highlights society's unwillingness to take IPV victims seriously and hold batterers accountable, especially within particular law enforcement organizations.

Chaney and Saltzstein (1998) stated that police department officials who disagree with current policies simply place their organizational efforts and resources in other areas, and in doing so, fail to provide the resources to train officers and therefore properly enforce IPV laws. Unfortunately, many courts have failed to hold officers and their respective police departments liable for failing to protect citizens against their abusers. In Connecticut, police departments were acquitted in civil suits where victims were falsely arrested (Martin, 1997). Cases against police departments in other states resulted in similar outcomes. In the case of *Eckert v. Town of Silverthorne* (2001), the victim claimed that the state of Colorado failed to train its police officers in properly protecting victims from violent batterers. The court, however, decided that the police officers were justified in arresting the victim under probable cause. In a similar case, *Welch v. City of New York* (1998), the victim accused a NYPD officer of false arrest and imprisonment. The court ultimately decided that the arrest was warranted, citing that the officer acted with probable cause and was entitled to qualified immunity.

As past history has shown, poor implementation of the law will not be curtailed without accountability for such failures from the courts (Finn et al., 2004). Officers can simply arrest both parties without proper investigation with little direct negative outcome (Martin, 1997; Miller, 2001). Thus, officers' inability to properly and effectively respond to IPV situations may be attributed to various factors, including poor training, individual beliefs and biases, and the overall lack of accountability.

If IPV victims were rarely arrested and thereby not entered into the criminal justice system, problems with prosecutors and judges would be a non-issue. This has led some authors to conclude that to effectively curb the problem of victim arrest, interventions should largely target those who make the decisions at the scene (i.e., police officers; Gardner, this issue; O'Dell, this issue). Nevertheless, once a victim enters the system, the potential for further abuses abound. Prosecutorial decisions such as failure to pursue indictments, prosecuting without victim consent, or forcing victim testimony under threat of arrest are also influenced by backlash forces (e.g., Bohmer et al., 2002; Mills, 1998, 1999). In addition, judges are notorious for their variability across jurisdictions in terms of case management, determinations concerning testimony and admission of evidence, and their overall viewpoints and biases about IPV (Brigner, 2003). And as shown above, recently our court systems have failed to hold police accountable for the false arrest of victims, allowing poor implementation at the scene to continue unabated.

Victims who are falsely arrested are often further disadvantaged by their lack of knowledge of the criminal justice system or its processes (Miller, 2001). Victims may be charged inappropriately, be falsely convicted, or even forced to plea bargain without being aware of their rights or options (Goodmark, 2004). They may also be coerced by prosecutors to testify or face the consequence of arrest for failing to do so, especially in jurisdictions that have implemented mandatory prosecution or no-drop policies (Goodmark). Judges may also order victims to attend treatment programs originally intended for and based on approaches for male primary batterers (Feder & Henning, 2005; Hamberger & Potente, 1994; Henning et al., 2006).

THE NEGATIVE EFFECTS OF VICTIM ARRESTS

Victims of IPV are already faced with many hardships as a result of violent partners. Many are now being labeled as the primary perpetrator as a result of increased victim arrests nationwide, even though it has been known for some time that women are overwhelmingly the victims of ongoing and severe IPV (Haviland et al., 2001; Henning & Feder, 2004), and as shown above, a review of studies to date shows that only about 1-7% of all women arrested for IPV are clearly primary perpetrators. Needless to say, falsely blaming and labeling the victim as an offender further deepens the lack of protection afforded to victims and potentially escalates the violence (Zorza, 1994).

As noted above, batterers will use the victim's IPV arrest to further control the situation. For example, a victim's prior history of arrest is used by some batterers to block the victim's attempt to press future criminal charges (Humphries, 2002), and batterers may maintain their control by threatening victims with further retaliatory charges (Goodmark, 2004). In addition, convictions have been used against victims in future court proceedings, particularly child custody cases (Goodmark). Furthermore, several states, including California, Illinois, Nebraska, and New York, have successfully removed children from violent homes, citing that the mother failed to protect her children from the batterer, while others have been charged with child endangerment due to the batterer's behavior and/or her own false arrest (Volovski, 2004).

In addition to the possibility of losing her children, victims falsely arrested are also liable to lose their jobs, often resulting in financial hardship. Such individuals are forced to call in sick or take leave in order to contest court charges, which often places their job security at risk, or may face employers who will not hire candidates with criminal records. The consequences are even more severe for victims who are immigrants because arrests or convictions can lead to deportation (Humphries, 2002). As a result, immigrant women are often forced to maintain a relationship that is violent or risk being returned to a country or family that may no longer accept them (Abraham, 2000).

Overall, the negative effects of erroneous arrest on victims are often overwhelming and long-term. Reports from victims reveal the negative impact of false arrest on their mental health, physical well-being, financial condition, family, and other personal relationships (Dutton & Goodman, 2005; Haviland et al., 2001; Henning et al., 2006). Erroneously arrested victims may report feelings of humiliation, exasperation, and the loss of will to continue to resist the violent behavior of the batterer (Hamberger & Potente, 1994). With the perpetuation of unjustified arrests, there will most probably be a decreasing number of victims willing to report incidents of IPV, or to otherwise turn to the criminal justice system for support and aid (Martin, 1997).

IMPLICATIONS AND RECOMMENDATIONS

From the previous discussion, it is apparent that the increase in victim arrest rates is not only a gross distortion of the intention and purpose of years of social change, but also poses a life-threatening risk for many women across the U.S. As such, it is imperative that further changes be enacted to contend with the weaknesses in current laws and statutes, failures in law enforcement, and the far-reaching social backlash we are currently experiencing.

One area of focus is previous statutes and laws concerning IPV. It is necessary for there to be clear guidelines on the proper police protocol at the IPV scene. As previously stated, the PPA statutes are failing to be either effective or fair. First, the PPA provision states that officers must assess the extent of injuries found on either party before making an arrest decision. Unfortunately, the types of injuries perpetrated by men and women are different and, as such, leave varying evidence of occurrence. Women typically inflict injuries that tend to appear immediately and visibly (i.e., scratches or bites). Men, on the other hand, perpetrate types of violence that may take days to appear, such as strangling (Klein, 2004). Thus, to base the arrest decision on immediate and visible injury could lead to the revictimization of those who were acting in self-defense. Although the PPA clearly states that officers are to determine if self-defense is present, it is evident from previous research that this is not occurring. In addition, savvy batterers can learn to manipulate the system by creating self-inflicted visible injuries as a means to control and threaten their partners (O'Dell, this issue). As such, it is important for future statutes to take these factors into consideration because they can prevent the false arrest of countless victims. Also, it cannot be stated strongly enough that the courts, across jurisdictions and states, should clearly be holding police departments and their officers accountable for the widespread increase in false arrests. Unfortunately, as noted above, this is not presently the case.

Another area of focus in preventing victim arrests is in the proper education of law enforcement and criminal justice officials. It is necessary for police officers, lawyers, and judges alike to be familiar with IPV and the context in which violence may occur. Included in this knowledge base are the complexities involved in IPV cases with respect to ongoing power dynamics within relationships, as well as the motivational factors behind the use of violence. If criminal justice officials are more knowledgeable about IPV cases, they may in turn be more willing to take the time to assess the situation carefully. In addition, if officers at the scene are able to access criminal records and previous IPV calls, it can help them make more reliable decisions regarding the primary batterer (Feder & Henning, 2005). Taken together, these factors may ameliorate any confusion during arrest or prosecution and can help prevent false arrests and convictions. Education may also increase the willingness of judges to hold police jurisdictions accountable for false IPV arrests.

As such, it may be helpful to have a domestic violence unit in police departments that consists of officers who are thoroughly trained concerning IPV situations. As Klein (2004) states, dual arrest rates have dropped in jurisdictions with proper police training and management. O'Dell (this issue), as well as Hamberger and Potente (1994), offer beneficial recommendations with regard to officer training and thus, these recommendations will not be repeated here. With respect to court cases, Brigner (2003) and Hamberger and Potente (1994) urge lawyers and judges to not only allow but also seek out expert testimony from individuals with experience in false victim arrests and victims' use of self-defense.

Training alone may not create large enough changes in officers' decisions to arrest both offenders and victims. Thus, it is important to recognize the role of masculinity and patriarchy on law enforcement officials' decision to arrest. As previous research shows, police officers are predominantly male themselves, and are thus apt to arrest women who do not fit the stereotype of the typical, subservient, and/or passive victim. Hence, a part of the change that must take place is in the traditional views officers hold. There also needs to be revisions in policies that are dominated by notions such as the "old boys' network," where women's concerns and issues are taken less seriously than men's. Consequently, criminal justice officials may operate under assumptions that women are to be obedient to their male partners and that men have the right to abuse their female partners to keep them in line. It is futile to pass laws that attempt to protect victims against false arrest if officers continue to work under stereotypical gender assumptions and therefore half-heartedly enforce the law at the scene.

Uniform implementation of investigative procedures across different jurisdictions is also important. With the creation of a uniform police protocol for use at the IPV scene, there will be fewer chances for confusion or erroneous arrests (see O'Dell, this issue). In addition, there should be support from all jurisdictions regarding the proper enforcement of IPV laws. As studies have shown, some officers are resentful of mandatory arrest laws, which they may believe strip them of their own discretionary powers. Uniform implementation and education may help alleviate these reactions, but it is essential for jurisdictions to first stand behind these policies at the top level and enforce officer adherence through clear consequences.

Another problematic outcome of the present backlash is the rates with which women are sent to batterer treatment programs designed for male batterers. As Gardner (this issue) and Hamberger and Potente (1994) state, women who are violent often become involved in a pattern of violence that they have not initiated or are able to control. As a result, the rates of recidivism for female aggressors are significantly lower when compared to their male counterparts. Despite such knowledge, women continue to be sent to treatment programs that were initially created for and directed at men (Henning & Renauer, 2005). As research has shown, such services may be inappropriate for women whose violent behavior is ultimately different from men (Hamberger, 2005a). Thus, services for women must take into account their specific needs and concerns, possibly including victimization services (Feder & Henning, 2005). In addition, programs can teach women about creating support networks that they can turn to in times of crisis, which may help some women to leave abusive situations (Hamberger, 2005b). Treatment services can also provide women with appropriate safety planning techniques (Dutton & Goodman, 2005). Additional recommendations include teaching women about their responsibility in committing aggressive acts, alternative solutions to violent situations, communication skills, frustration tolerance, and socially appropriate assertiveness (Dutton & Goodman).

Along with the focus on the criminal justice system, it is important to realize the impact of research on legislation and other social policy. As the Minneapolis Domestic Violence Experiment once promoted changes in the early 1980's, research can clearly influence shifts in IPV policy. However, research-driven policy shifts can be detrimental depending on the scientific methodology on which these studies are based. Over the past decades, decontexualized research results highlighting gender symmetry and equality in IPV have led to not only the increased support and visibility of men's rights activists, but have also potentially led to the loss of much needed resources from battered women's programs. They have also slowed, if not stopped, coordinated community batterer accountability efforts. It is also important to recognize that many of the studies that have found equivalent rates of violence among men and women, and even those studies showing higher rates among women, suffer from numerous methodological weaknesses. Such gender-symmetric findings are limited to only those approaches, such as the CTS, that decontextualize IPV and reflect little of the fear, threats, psychological harm, severe injuries, and repeated victimization experienced by women who are now losing funding and potential resources. To publish such decontextualized and thus methodologically poor studies that show IPV is predominantly gender symmetrical is not only superfluous, it approaches negligence. These types of methodologically unsound and widely criticized studies do little to hold batterers accountable and are instead used for just the opposite effect. Thus, it is our responsibility to be clear in our research methodology and even clearer when stating our findings. It is essential to reproduce previous findings on the perpetration of IPV using advanced measurement tools and frameworks that incorporate multiple contextual factors, such as ongoing coercion and control (Brush, 2005). It is also essential that research findings concerning the increase of false victim arrests be widely disseminated and used to advocate for societal change, and that researchers never lose sight of the fact that they, too, are susceptible to societal backlash influences.

In summary, whether it arises from patriarchal ideals, stereotypical assumptions of gender roles, or issues concerning power and control, IPV is a reality in our society. Despite years of work and change, victims of IPV face continued struggles searching for safety and justice not only from their abusers, but from researchers and the criminal justice system as well. Confusion over IPV laws and policies within the criminal justice system has led to an increase in the number of victim arrests. These rising rates have been used by male rights activists and others as evidence that women are as violent, or even more so, than men. Such beliefs have prompted multiple studies examining gender differences in the perpetration of IPV, some of which conclude that IPV rates are equivalent, and at times even higher, among women. Thus, it is important for future research to be conducted that is contextualized and measures ongoing patterns of IPV. These future studies may then help form new IPV policies and laws that can benefit victims and hold batterers accountable. In doing so, greater resources may be available to hold

batterers accountable in order to deliver swift consequences for breaking the law. If not, victims of IPV will continue to lose faith in the system and face an increasing number of negative consequences in the
legal, financial, physical health, and psychological realms, while
batterers will continue to abuse with impunity.

REFERENCES

Abraham, M. (2000). *Speaking the unspeakable: Marital violence among South Asian
immigrants in the United States.* New Brunswick, NJ: Rutgers University Press.
Anderson, K. L. (2005). Theorizing gender in intimate partner violence research. *Sex
Roles: A Journal of Research, 52*(11-12), 853-866.
Bachman, R., & Coker, A. L. (1995). Police involvement in domestic violence: The in-
teractive effects of victim injury, offender's history of violence, and race. *Violence
and Victims, 10*(2), 91-106.
Belknap, J. (1995). Law enforcement officers' attitudes about the appropriate re-
sponses to woman battering. *International Review of Victimology, 4*(1), 47-62.
Bennett, L., Goodman, L., & Dutton, M. (1999). Systemic obstacles to the criminal
prosecution of a battering partner: A victim perspective. *Journal of Interpersonal
Violence, 14*(7), 761-772.
Berk, R. A., Campbell, A., Klap, R., & Western, B. (1992). The deterrent effect of arrest in incidents of domestic violence: A Bayesian analysis of four field experi-
ments. *American Sociological Review, 57*(5), 698-708.
Bible, A., Dasgupta, S., & Osthoff, S. (Eds.) (2002-2003). Women's use of violence in
intimate relationships: Part 1, 2, 3 [Special issues]. *Violence Against Women,
8*(11-12), 9(1).
Bohmer, C., Brandt, J., Bronson, D., & Hartnett, H. (2002). Domestic violence law reforms: Reactions from the trenches. *Journal of Sociology and Social Welfare,
29*(3), 71-86.
Bourg, S., & Stock, H. (1994). A review of domestic violence arrest statistics in a police department using a pro-arrest policy: Are pro-arrest policies enough? *Journal
of Family Violence, 9*(2), 177-183.
Boyle, K. (2005). *Media and violence.* Thousand Oaks, CA: Sage Publications.
Brigner, M. (2003). *The Ohio domestic violence benchbook: A practical guide to com-
petence for judges and magistrates* (2nd ed.). Columbus, OH: Family Violence Prevention Center at the Ohio Office of Criminal Justice Services.
Bruno v. Codd, 64 A.D.2d 582; 407 N.Y.S.2d165 (1978).
Brush, L. D. (2005). Philosophical and political issues in research on women's violence and aggression. *Sex Roles: A Journal of Research, 52*(11-12), 867-874.
Buttell, F. P., & Carney, M. M. (Eds.) (2006). *Women who perpetrate relationship violence: Moving beyond political correctness.* Binghamton, NY: Haworth Press.
Buzawa, E. S., & Buzawa, C. G. (2003). *Domestic violence: The criminal justice re-
sponse.* Thousand Oaks, CA: Sage.

Carlson, C., & Nidey, F. (1995). Mandatory penalties, victim cooperation, and the judicial processing of domestic abuse cases. *Crime and Delinquency, 41*(1), 132-149.

Chaney, C., & Saltzstein, G. (1998). Democratic control and bureaucratic responsiveness: The police and domestic violence. *American Journal of Political Science, 42*(3), 745-768.

Chesney-Lind, M. (2002). Criminalizing victimization: The unintended consequences of pro-arrest policies for girls and women. *Criminology and Public Policy, 2*(1), 81-91.

Chesney-Lind, M., & Pasko, L. (2004). *The female offender: Girls, women, and crime.* Thousand Oaks, CA: Sage.

Cook, S., L., & Swan, S. C. (Eds.) (2006). Special issue. *Violence Against Women, 12*(11).

Danis, F. S. (2003). The criminalization of domestic violence: What social workers need to know. *Social Work, 48*(2), 237-247.

Dasgupta, S. (2003) *Safety and justice for all: Examining the relationship between the women's anti-violence movement and the criminal justice system.* New York: Ms Foundation.

DeKeseredy, W. S. (1999). Tactics of the antifeminist backlash against Canadian national woman abuse surveys. *Violence Against Women, 5*(11), 1258-1276.

Dowd, L. S., Leisring, P. A., & Rosenbaum, A. (2005). Partner aggressive women: Characteristics and treatment attrition. *Violence and Victims, 20*(2), 219-231.

Dugan, L. (2003). Domestic violence legislation: Exploring its impact on the likelihood of domestic violence, police involvement, and arrest. *Criminology and Public Policy, 2*(2), 283-312.

Dutton, M. A., & Goodman, L. A. (2005). Coercion in intimate partner violence: Toward a new conceptualization. *Sex Roles: A Journal of Research, 52*(11-12), 743-757.

Eckert v. Town of Silverthorne, 25 Fed. Appx. 679 (Colo. Ct. App. 2001).

Fagan, J. A. (1996). *The criminalization of domestic violence: Promises and limits.* Washington, DC: U.S. Department of Justice, Office of Justice Programs.

Family Violence Reporting Program. (1991). *Study of violence incidents which result in arrest of both parties.* Meriden, CT: Connecticut Department of Public Safety.

Feder, L. (1998). Police handling of domestic violence calls: Is there a case for discrimination? *Crime and Delinquency, 44*(2), 335-350.

Feder, L., & Henning, K. (2005). A comparison of male and female dually arrested domestic violence offenders. *Violence & Victims, 20*(2), 153-171.

Finn, M., Blackwell, B. S., Stalans, L. J., Studdard, S., & Dugan, L. (2004). Dual arrest decisions in domestic violence cases: The influence of departmental policies. *Crime and Delinquency, 50*(4), 565-589.

Fox, J. A., & Zawitz, M. W. (2006). *Homicide trends in the United States.* Washington, DC: U.S. Department of Justice, Bureau of Justice Statistics. Retrieved December 27, 2006 from, http://www.ojp.usdoj.gov/bjs/homicide/intimates.htm

Frieze, I. H., & McHugh, M. C. (Eds.) (2005). Special issue: Female violence against intimate partners. *Psychology of Women Quarterly, 29*(3).

Gardner, D. (2007). Victim-defendants in mandated treatment: An ethical quandary. *Journal of Aggression, Maltreatment & Trauma, 15*(3/4), 75-93.

Geffner, R., Sorenson, S. B., & Lundbger-Love, P. K. (1997). *Violence and sexual abuse at home: Current issues in spousal battering and child maltreatment.* New York: Haworth.

Goodmark, L. (2004). The legal response to domestic violence: Problems and possibilities: Law is the answer? Do we know that for sure? Questioning the efficacy of legal interventions for battered women. *Saint Louis University Public Law Review, 7,* 1-46.

Groves v. State University of New York, No. 86119, 2000 N.Y. App. Div., 265 A.D.2d 141, 707 N.Y.S.2d 261, LEXIS 4430, at *2-3 (A.D. NY April 20, 2000).

Hamberger, K. L. (2005a). Men's and women's use of intimate partner violence in clinical samples: Toward a gender sensitive analysis. *Violence and Victims, 20*(2), 131-151.

Hamberger, L. K. (Ed.) (2005b). Special issue on men's and women's use of intimate partner violence. *Violence and Victims, 20*(3).

Hamberger, K., & Potente, T. (1994). Counseling heterosexual women arrested for domestic violence: Who presents the greater threat? *Violence & Victims, 19*(2), 69-80.

Hamby, S. L. (2005). Measuring gender differences in partner violence: Implications from research on other forms of violence and socially undesirable behavior. *Sex Roles, 52*(11-12), 725-743.

Hartman, J., & Belknap, J. (2003). Beyond the gatekeepers: Court professionals' self reported attitudes about and experiences with domestic violence cases. *Criminal Justice and Behavior, 30*(3), 349-373.

Haviland, M., Frye V., Rajah, V., Thukral, J. & Trinity, M. (2001). *The Family Protection and Domestic Violence Intervention Act of 1995: Examining the effects of mandatory arrest in New York City.* New York: Urban Justice Center.

Henning, K., & Feder, L. (2004). A comparison of men and women arrested for domestic violence: Who presents the greater threat? *Journal of Family Violence, 19*(2), 69-80.

Henning, K., & Renauer, B. (2005). Prosecution of women arrested for intimate partner abuse. *Violence & Victims, 20*(3), 361-375.

Henning, K., Renauer, B., & Holdford, R. (2006). Victim or offender? Heterogeneity among women arrested for intimate partner violence. *Journal of Family Violence, 21*(6), 351-368.

Hirschel, J. D., Hutchison, I. W., Dean, C. W., & Mills, A. (1992). Review essay on the law enforcement response to spouse abuse: Past, present and future. *Justice Quarterly, 9,* 247-83.

Humphries, D. (2002). No easy answers: Public policy, criminal justice, and domestic violence. *Criminology & Public Policy, 2*(1), 91-96.

Kim, M. (2004). *The community engagement continuum: Outreach, mobilization, organizing and accountability to address violence against women in Asian and Pacific Islander communities.* San Francisco, CA: Asian & Pacific Islander Institute on Domestic Violence.

Klein, A. R. (2004). *The criminal justice system response to domestic violence.* Belmont, CA: Wadsworth.

Library of Congress. (1994). *H.R.3355: Violent Crime Control and Law Enforcement Act of 1994 - Title IV. Violence Against Women.* Washington DC: Author. Retrieved June 1, 2007 from, http://thomas.loc.gov/cgi-bin/query/z?c103:H.R.3355.ENR:

Malloy, K. A., McCloskey, K. A., Grigsby, N., & Gardner, D. (2003). Women's use of violence within intimate relationships. *Journal of Aggression, Maltreatment, and Trauma, 6*(2), 37-59.

Martin, M. E. (1997). Double your trouble: Dual arrest in family violence. *Journal of Family Violence, 12*(2), 139-157.

Maxwell, C., Garner, J., & Fagan, J. (2002). The preventive effects of arrest on intimate partner violence: Research, policy and theory. *Criminology & Public Policy, 2*(1), 51-80.

McHugh, M. C., & Frieze, I. H. (Eds.) (2005). Special issue: Understanding gender and intimate partner violence: Theoretical and empirical approaches. *Sex Roles, 52*(11-12).

Men's Rights. (n.d.). *Domestic violence.* Retrieved September 5, 2006 from, http://en.wikipedia.org/wiki/Men%27s_rights#Violence

Middap, C. (2000). *Gloves off in battle of sexes: Domestic violence–abusive women.* Retrieved September 5, 2006 from, www.mensrights.com.au/index.php?menu_cd =dmv&cat_cd=awm

Mignon, S. I., & Holmes, W. M. (1995). Police response to mandatory arrest laws. *Crime and Delinquency, 41*(4), 430-442.

Miller, S. L. (2001). The paradox of women arrested for domestic violence: Criminal justice professionals and service providers respond. *Violence Against Women, 7*(12), 1339-1376.

Mills, L. G. (1998). Mandatory arrest and prosecution policies for domestic violence. *Criminal Justice and Behavior, 25*(3), 306-318.

Mills, L. G. (1999). Killing her softly: Intimate abuse and the violence of state interventions. *Harvard Law Review, 113*, 550-613.

O'Dell, A. (2007). Why do police arrest victims of domestic violence? The need for comprehensive training and investigative protocols. *Journal of Aggression, Maltreatment & Trauma, 15*(3/4), 53-73.

Paulozzi, L. J., Saltzman, L. E., Thompson, M. P., & Holmgreen, P. (2001). Surveillance for homicide among intimate partners - United States, 1981-1998. *Morbidity and Mortality Weekly Report, 50*(SS03), 1-6.

Pennsylvania Supreme Court Committee on Racial and Gender Bias. (2003). Domestic violence, Chapter 10. In *Final report of the Pennsylvania Supreme Court Committee on Racial and Gender Bias in the justice system* (pp. 385-418). Harrisburg, PA: Pennsylvania Judicial Center.

Renzetti, C. M. (1996). On dancing with a bear: Reflections on some of the current debates among domestic violence theorists. In L. K. Hamberger & C. M. Renzetti (Eds.), *Domestic partner abuse* (pp. 213-222). New York: Springer.

Robinson, A. L., & Chandek, M. S. (2000). Differential police response to black battered women. *Women and Criminal Justice, 12*(2/3), 29-61.

Saunders, D. G. (1995). The tendency to arrest victims of domestic violence: A preliminary analysis of officer characteristics. *Journal of Interpersonal Violence, 10*, 147-58.

Sitaker, M. (2007). The ecology of intimate partner violence: Theorized impacts on women's use of violence. *Journal of Aggression, Maltreatment & Trauma, 15*(3/4), 179-219.

State of California Office of the Attorney General. (1999). Report on arrests for domestic violence in California, 1998. *Criminal Justice Statistics Center Report Series, 1(3),* 1-21.

State of New York. (1998). *Family Protection and Domestic Violence Intervention Act of 1994: Evaluation of the mandatory arrest provisions–Interim report to the Governor and the Legislature, January 1997.* Albany, NY: State of New York Division of Criminal Justice Services, Office for the Prevention of Domestic Violence.

Steinmetz, S. K., & Straus, M. A. (1974). *Violence in the family.* New York: Dodd, Mead.

Straus, M. A. (2004). Prevalence of violence against dating partners by male and female university students worldwide. *Violence Against Women, 10*(7), 790-811.

Straus, M. A. (2005, July). *Gender and partner violence in world perspective: Results from the International Dating Violence Study.* Paper presented at the University of New Hampshire International Family Violence Research Conference, Portsmouth, NH.

Straus, M. A. (2006). Future research on gender symmetry in physical assaults on partners. *Violence Against Women, 12*(11), 1086-1097.

Straus, M. A., & Gelles, R. J. (1986). Societal change and change in family violence from 1975 to 1985 as revealed by two national surveys. *Journal of Marriage and the Family, 48*(3), 465-479.

Swan, S., & Snow, D. (2002). A typology of women's use of violence in intimate relationships. *Violence Against Women, 8*(3), 286-319.

Thurman v. City of Torrington, 595 F. Supp. 1521 (1984).

Volovski, K. E. (2004). Domestic violence. *The Georgetown Journal of Gender and the Law, Spring, 175/S,* 124-130.

Welch v. City of New York, No. 98-7533, U.S. App. (1998).

World Health Organization. (2005). *WHO multi-country study on women's health and domestic violence against women.* Geneva, Switzerland: Author.

Zorza, J. (1994). Must we stop arresting batterers? Analysis and policy implications of new police domestic violence studies. *New England Law Review, 28,* 929-990.

Submitted: January 19, 2007
Revised: April 6, 2007
Revised: June 1, 2007
Accepted: June 3, 2007

Why Do Police Arrest Victims of Domestic Violence? The Need for Comprehensive Training and Investigative Protocols

Anne O'Dell

Between October 1975 and October 1995, I worked as a police officer and sergeant/supervisor on the San Diego Police Department. During that time, I worked in some fashion on over 70,000 cases of domestic violence (DV). In the last nine years, I have traveled internationally and nationally both training others and being trained on DV and stalking. I have had occasion to meet and speak extensively with survivors, victims, abusers, and various law enforcement, medical, and judicial personnel, and have heard their stories. In this article, I will cover the mistakes that law enforcement officers have repeatedly made (and still make) when arresting individuals for DV. I will also cover what they can do to consistently correct these deficiencies. Why these mistakes are made will be discussed, as well as suggestions for specific training designed to help officers more accurately determine the suspect at the scene.

THE CONTEXT:
A SHORT HISTORY
OF THE CRIMINAL JUSTICE RESPONSE
TO DOMESTIC VIOLENCE

A short history of how the laws in the U.S. have reflected the issue of DV first seems warranted. While an exhaustive historical treatment is not the topic of this article and has been accomplished elsewhere (e.g., Erez, 2002; Pleck, 1987; Worden, 2000; Zorza, 1992), it is important to present a short review in order to provide a relevant context for the following discussion. Historically, violence against women in intimate relationships was not considered a crime; indeed, as recently as 1979, case law upheld the right of a male head of household to physically chastise and otherwise punish his wife unless some lasting physical injury was inflicted (Erez). Social change movements in the 1970s, as well as legal action against police units that failed to protect women from severe injury and even death at the hands of their male partners, created a present-day situation where virtually every state has passed laws against DV at least at the level of a misdemeanor offense (Erez; Worden). Corresponding to these changes in the law, three distinct yet overlapping phases in the evolution of police response to DV have been documented: (a) the *traditional response*: before the mid-1970s, police separated the parties for a "cool down" period with no subsequent arrests; (b) the *service response*: in the 1970s to the mid-1980s, police were trained in DV issues, provided parties with social service contacts, and made arrests based on judgments at the scene; and (c) the *mandatory/preferred arrest response*: from the 1980s to the present, many police are now required by law or otherwise pressured by criminal justice administrators in their jurisdictions to make an arrest at the DV scene (Breci, 2002; Erez, 2002).

While a discussion of the strengths and weaknesses of the three phases given above is beyond the scope of this article (and have been addressed elsewhere: see Breci, 2002; Erez, 2002; Melton, 1999; Stewart, 2001), they are nevertheless illustrative of the social changes occurring in the last 30 years. However, as with any social change that becomes institutionalized, legislative changes tend to be ahead of both personal belief structures and correct implementation of those changes within the community (Robinson, 2000; Stith, 1990). It should not be surprising, then, that police officers do not always implement the "spirit of the law" at the scene, especially with mandatory/preferred arrest scenarios.

ISSUES SURROUNDING ILLEGAL ARREST OF VICTIMS

Police Culture

In many ways, police agencies found in local communities resemble a paramilitary and patriarchal culture. For instance, hierarchical structures as well as weapons and combat training are inculcated within these agencies, very similar to that found in U.S. military structures. In addition, it is no secret that police work tends to attract mostly men to its ranks, also quite similar to the military. These two components, the presence of a paramilitary structure/mindset coupled with a predominantly male workforce, can easily create a situation wherein thrill-seeking, normative violent behavior, and bragging about sexual conquests are commonplace. These types of behaviors were labeled "hypermasculine" by Mosher and colleagues in the 1980s and have been linked to many different types of predominantly male groups, including military-type units (Mosher & Sirkin, 1984; Mosher & Tomkins, 1988). A correlate of hypermasculinity is "hostile masculinity," wherein men endorse domination and control over women, including the use of violent behavior to enforce that dominance. Murnen, Wright, and Kaluzny (2002) found that attitudes endorsing dominance over and hostility towards women strongly predicted self-reported perpetration of sexual violence.

Some studies examining male police officers' beliefs about gender roles and attitudes have shown that they do endorse many rigidly masculine beliefs (Robinson, 2000; Robinson & Chandek, 2000; Stith, 1990), but that the link between self-reported gender role adherence and actual response to DV victims and perpetrators at the scene is still largely unknown and unexplored. However, given the coupling of a military-type structure with a predominantly male workforce, it is not unreasonable to suggest that some of the problems related to arresting victims at the scene may be influenced by officers' personal beliefs in many masculine stereotypes that support hostility toward women. Given that victims of DV are overwhelmingly female, male officers may often have little understanding of DV from a victim's perspective. Furthermore, changes in domestic violence laws may create resentment and frustration within the ranks, and be perceived as unwelcome and arbitrarily imposed social engineering. As seen below, gender stereotypes and lack of understanding on the part of officers can adversely impact the implementation of mandatory/preferred arrest policies within the community.

The Myth of Mutual Combat

There is little true mutual combat in DV cases. Contrary to popular mythology, it does not "take two to tango" within domestic violence cases. By its very definition of power and control, violence, intimidation, and patterned history, mutual combat is rare in DV relationships (Hamberger, 1997; Malloy, McCloskey, Grigsby, & Gardner, 2003; Miller, 2001), and many males who claim to be victimized by their female partners are perpetrators in prior arrests (Muelleman & Burgess, 1998). True mutual combat could be described as two men in a bar of equal size, ability, and capacity to inflict injury on one another and with no history of previous intimate relationship or power and control issues. A prosecutor colleague describes it as "Tombstone Corral" at high noon, where two cowboys stand back-to-back, walk away from each other, and at 20 steps then turn and shoot at each other in a duel.

Informal observations at the San Diego Police Department suggest that an acceptable rate of mutual combat arrests is a maximum of about 3% of all DV-related arrests. This observation is based, in aggregate, on the many actual DV investigative reports that were later deemed inaccurate and had resulted in erroneous arrests (see below). These informal observations are in line with recent research results. For example, Henning, Renauer, and Holdford (2006) reported that 485 females represented 13% of all clients (about 3,730) court-ordered for an IPV perpetrator assessment, and of these 485 women, only 9% (about 30) could be clearly identified as the primary aggressor, with approximately 35% of the women not falling cleanly into either a perpetrator or victim category. From that data set, it seems that only 30 of the identified 3,730 clients referred for assessment (less than 1%) could clearly be identified as a female primary aggressor. Even with a more liberal application of Henning, Renauer, and Holdford's classification scheme using the 35% estimate of unclassified females, only about 4.5% of the entire sample of 3,730 could reasonably be thought of as female primary perpetrators. Thus, according to the above results, an acceptable rate lies somewhere between 1%-5%. Similarly, Klein (2004) found that even within the same state, police practices and therefore dual arrests and arrests of females vary widely. He cited dual arrests rates ranging from a low of 1.9% in Providence, Rhode Island to a high of 25% in Warwick, Rhode Island. He also noted that "East Providence's 13.5% dual arrest rate plummeted in 2000, for example, to 3.2% the next year, from 33 to 8 arrests, largely because of the reassignment of a single superior officer charged with the night shift" (p. 109). Klein reported that while many jurisdictions have seen whopping increases in female arrests in general (e.g., a 511% increase in arrests of women between 1988 and 2001 compared to an increase of 143% for men in the state of California), other jurisdictions "have gradually reduced both dual and female arrests through training and police management" (p. 109). He reported that dual arrests declined to about 6% in Lincoln, Nebraska through targeted training. Unfortunately, there are still many law enforcement agencies that make mutual combat arrests in much higher percentages (from a high of about 22% in Connecticut to a low of about 1% in Oklahoma; Klein). If a jurisdiction or a law enforcement agency has a percentage higher than 1% to 6%, it most probably indicates a lack of good training or a clear policy to direct officers properly in DV investigations (see the discussion below). It also indicates an insufficient or inadequate investigation.

Officers in my DV training classes complain that supervisors do not always allow them the time to stay at the crime scene to conduct a proper and complete investigation. An example of a good policy that prevents mutual combat arrests is to require the arresting officer to justify the probable cause of each arrest independently in separate reports. The mandate to write two complete reports sometimes motivates officers to spend the requisite time necessary to clearly identify the suspect and the victim.

In my experience, sometimes an officer may want to believe that whoever strikes the first blow or throws the first item is the primary aggressor. During training, we often use scenarios in which an officer must react in a pre-emptive way with aggressive actions against a suspect, or risk being hurt. Officers must use different levels of self-defense based on the suspect's actions, and are legally justified in doing so. We then compare the officers' justified use of force to that of a battered woman's use of force in her own home.

In addition, most officers are perfectly able to determine who should go to jail for a criminal assault and who has inflicted injury during an assault. In virtually every state, sections of assault laws typically include words like "intentional, reckless, and/or willful." Those actions are obviously *not* actions in self-defense. All officers need to do to overcome the tendency to arrest both the victim and perpetrator at a DV scene is complete a proper criminal investigation, just as they are required to do at any other assault scene. I often challenge officers who see a DV incident as "murky" or "confusing" during training sessions to consider how they would want their Internal Affairs detectives to investigate their *own* use of force at an incident scene.

Even the holding and pointing of a weapon by a woman does not necessarily constitute an assault or violation of the law. One needs to examine the context in which it happens. There is a large difference between the following two scenarios. In the first scenario, a woman with a history of being battered is in her home when her husband returns. He is drunk and obnoxious, which is typical of his behavior when he has battered her in the past. She is well aware of exactly how he acts just before he hits her. She retreats to the kitchen as his behavior escalates. He follows and begins to threaten her with body language and/or words. She backs up to a drawer, pulls out a knife, and tells him to stay away. Question: "Threatening with a weapon or an attempt to protect oneself?" In the second scenario, a woman with no history of abuse is in her home. Her drunken husband comes home and she begins to berate him for drinking. She then gets a knife in the kitchen and begins to threaten him with it. Question: "Threatening with a weapon or an attempt to protect oneself?"

There is obviously a huge difference between the above situations. It depends on the context in which things happen as well as the history between the individuals. One of the earliest studies in the U.S. concerning historical factors showed that violence between intimates was highly repetitive (Wilson, 1977); for previous assaults and homicides in a two year period, police had been called to the scene at least once in 85% of the cases, and five times or more in half of the cases.

When we now train officers, we draw correlations between the officer's right to defend him- or herself from imminent threat, as well as any other citizen's right to do the same as protected under the U.S. constitution: that is, the right to be free from physical harm. This strategy also helps us to more easily explain who the "primary" aggressor is in what may first appear to be "mutual combat."

In summary, masculine ideology and structure within police agencies, prevailing myths concerning mutual combat, and a lack of training in DV issues from a victim's perspective all contribute to illegal arrests of victims at the scene. It seems evident that enough time should be allotted to officers to conduct a thorough investigation, effective interviewing techniques should be used, an appropriate history and all available evidence should be collected from all parties, every witness who heard or saw anything should be interviewed, and the subsequent report should be properly and thoroughly completed. When this approach is used, officers usually have little problem determining who the primary aggressor is and whether self-defense is an issue. Finally, when we decide to train officers on how to recognize self-defense and how to distinguish protective violence from mutual combat, we also need to include the thorny, controversial issues of male privilege and entitlement, as well as the officer's own history, biases, and agendas. The harsh reality is that false arrests of victims defending themselves are made routinely when we fail to train officers appropriately.

WHAT POLICE DO WRONG:
MISTAKES AT THE SCENE

Specific Case Studies from San Diego

I first discovered our inadequacies in arresting the correct suspect at DV scenes in 1992. The San Diego Police Department's DV Investigations Unit had just been established and staffed. Thirty two candidates had vied for positions in the new unit. Of these, 16 detectives had been selected along with 2 sergeants, 1 lieutenant, and various support staff. The unit was open seven days a week. This made perfect sense, as nearly 35% of all our DV arrests were made between Friday night and Sunday night.

Maria and Jose. As 1 of the 2 sergeants assigned to the unit, I offered to work the weekends. Subsequently, on my first Saturday in the new unit, I arrived at 5:30 a.m. to prepare the cases for the "skeleton crew" of seven detectives scheduled to work that day. Part of my preparatory work with the DV cases included checking the criminal history background of each named suspect and attaching this information to cases before the detectives started their work. I also ran each suspect's name through our computer system, the Automated Regional Justice Information System (ARJIS). I checked the first dozen suspects through ARJIS and then started working on a case that involved a female as the suspect. She had been arrested on a felony charge of DV. She had no prior history of law enforcement contact within the ARJIS system. I began to read her arrest report.

Maria (not her real name) had finished her shift as a bartender at an East San Diego bar at 10 p.m. Friday night in late summer of 1992. She had decided to have a beer with two of the bar's patrons. She was sitting at a small table with the two men when her common law husband, Jose, (not his real name) walked into the bar with Maria's 15 year old son. Jose told Maria, "I'm here to take you home, Maria. Let's go." Maria told Jose to let her finish her beer. He objected and demanded she leave immediately. When she refused, he put down her beer, grabbed her from behind under her shoulders, and dragged her out of the bar. As she twisted around in an effort to get away from Jose, she scratched his cheek leaving two small scratches. When our local San Diego police responded, they "quickly assessed the situation" and, seeing two scratches on Jose's face, arrested Maria.

As I reviewed the report the next morning, I had the disturbing thought that I was reading the narrative of an illegal arrest. However, not wanting to make an arbitrary decision about it, when I routinely assigned the report to a detective I also included the comment that I had problems with the legality of the arrest. My intention was to have our regularly assigned prosecutor review the case on Monday morning to see if my early perception was correct. Monday morning came and the prosecutor reviewed the case. The prosecutor immediately asked me, "What the hell did our guys arrest her for?" I had to admit that none of us had included a component on how to recognize self-defense in our prior DV police training, and I personally felt responsible for this failure.

The prosecutor stated that this was a "bad arrest" and we should release Maria. The detective, who was standing there, disagreed with both of us and said that it was indeed a good arrest. When I questioned the detective, he explained his position by saying that the narrative written by the patrol officer clearly stated that Jose "only dragged her out of the bar because she was an alcoholic and he didn't want her drinking." When I challenged his reasoning by pointing out that nowhere in the California Penal Code did it state that husbands can drag their alcoholic wives out of bars, he continued by saying, "I used to be married to an alcoholic. I would have done the same damn thing." Disturbingly, this detective was a veteran officer with about 12 years in law enforcement.

I was astonished at his reasoning. At the time, though, I did not fully understand the problem. I later realized what the detective was saying: in his opinion, officers were allowed to inject issues such as male privilege and entitlement as well as personal bias and history into decisions about who goes to jail. Nevertheless, Maria was subsequently released from jail and her common-law husband, Jose, was then arrested.

Head banging, bite marks, and arresting the victim. One week later, another questionable case came into the DV Unit, one in which the "victim" (male, 6', 225 lbs.) suffered a bite mark to his chest. The "perpetrator" (female, 5'6", 135 lbs.) had no obvious injuries and was subsequently arrested on DV charges. The arresting patrol officers had seen the case as a "slam dunk." However, the case was undone and she was "un-arrested" once the DV Unit detective learned that the male in this case had straddled the woman, banged her head into the floor numerous times, and upon one particular bounce of her head she bit his chest in order to get free of his grip.

It quickly became apparent that some of our officers were rushing to judgment at the scene, as well as using only a part of the California state law's verbiage on DV assault, not the entire section. In one respect, our officers were trying to follow the new protocol on pro-arrest for DV. Officers would often state they were afraid *not* to make an arrest in DV situations. However, it soon became clear that our officers were reacting very quickly to the part of the law that states "any traumatic condition of the body, whether minor or major" is probable cause for arrest. However, they were ignoring the part of the law that states an assault is defined as "intentional, reckless, and/or willful." It also appeared that the concept of self-defense, a Constitutional right due the 14th Amendment, was largely being ignored in DV cases by officers at the scene. Ignorance surrounding this concept was apparent in spite of the fact that officers are very well versed in self-defense as it applied to themselves in their roles as police officers. As supervisors, we had our work cut out for us: it was time to train officers on how to recognize self-defense in DV cases.

Self-defensive "red flags." We began studying prior DV cases that included one party who acted in true self-defense, and learned there are common "red flags" in these cases. Then we began teaching officers these red flags, which mostly manifest as injuries on males in heterosexual partnerships. These injuries included scratches and/or bite marks on men's chests, arms, and/or legs. Scratches to men occur because women's fingernails are often an "equalizer." Most women are ill-equipped to successfully fight male partners on an equal physical level, and conversely, most men are not intimidated by the physical presence of a woman. In a physical attack, women are very likely to scratch their aggressor as a way to deflect attack or escape injury. Scratches are also a common injury when a woman is being strangled. Consider this case: a man is standing in front of a woman, strangling her with both hands. She is panicking and thinking she is about to die, an obviously credible belief since strangulation is a life threatening assault (Funk & Schuppel, 2003; Wilbur et al., 2001). She has both hands free. Most victims will instinctively claw an attacker's face to escape more serious injury or death. Add to this the fact that less than 20% of the time will there any be visible injuries on the woman's neck and/or throat; usually, there will be only internal injuries to the victim (Funk & Schuppel; Hawley, McClane, & Strack, 2001; McClane, Strack, & Hawley, 2001; Smith, Mills, & Taliaferro, 2001; Strack, McClane, & Hawley, 2001). Often, if the responding patrol officer has not been trained concerning the symptoms and identification of internal damage due to strangulation, the victim goes to jail. In addition, bite marks occur on males usually because their victims are in close proximity during an assault. Bites to the chest occur when a man is holding a woman down, straddling her, holding her in a bear hug, or sometimes during a sexual assault. Bite marks on the arms occur when the woman is being held in a chokehold or arm lock. It is not typical for a woman to run up to a man, hold his arm up, and bite underneath it (e.g., Pretty & Sweet, 2000). These types of injuries to a perpetrator are also known as "defensive injuries." Eventually it became clear that bite marks and scratches are strongly associated with defensive injuries in strangulation cases. Another type of defensive injury is to the male genital area. During investigations, we often found that male suspects were trying to force oral copulation and victims defended themselves by scratching, tearing, or biting the genitals of the suspect.

Sexual assault: "Swabbing a suspect's fingers." A colleague who is a DV unit sergeant in Delaware told me this story about an incident that happened in his department. This particular sergeant was on-call on a Sunday when he received a telephone call from a new officer. The rookie told the sergeant that he had two people in custody for DV. He further stated that he had completed a records search but found no prior information on either person. He said that both the male and female were close in size and both had equal types of injuries. Knowing that his agency frowned on dual arrests, the officer asked the sergeant to come to the station to assist him.

The sergeant arrived at the station to find the male and female in separate holding cells. The officer told the sergeant that the male had sustained bite marks and scratches on his body and the female had sustained bruises to her neck and the inside of one thigh. The sergeant started his investigation by interviewing the female. The female told him that she had been living with and dating "John" (not his real name) for about a year but that she was getting sick of the relationship. She said John was trying to control her, degraded her verbally, and was drinking more and more. Despite the fact that the female had asked John to get counseling, he had refused. She told the sergeant that she had gone out with a girlfriend on Saturday night and then decided to stay at the girlfriend's apartment overnight. She had discussed her problems about her relationship at length with her friend and by Sunday morning she had decided to leave John. When she had arrived at the house and walked into the living room, she said John had immediately confronted her by screaming and accusing her of "screwing around" on him. She tried to tell him that she had been with her best friend, but John said he did not believe her because her friend would lie for her anyway. The woman had finally told John that "enough was enough" and she was leaving because the relationship was not working out. As she turned and walked into the bedroom, John came up behind her and threw her to the bed. He then pulled off her pants while holding her by the neck. He then "checked her" to see if she had had sex with another man. While she was trying to get away from him, she scratched and bit him. The sergeant asked if anything else had happened. The woman stated that she was screaming loudly and someone had called the police.

The sergeant then went into the other holding cell to interview the man. The man's story was quite different. He told the sergeant his girlfriend had stayed out all night without calling him. He went on to state that when she finally came home, he had been very angry with her and accused her of cheating. The man said that when he accused her of cheating, the woman had "gone crazy" and starting scratching and biting him. The sergeant asked him again to reiterate his statement, which the man did. Finally, the sergeant recounted the story that the woman had told him. The male suspect was horrified and told the sergeant he would never do that, and further said that the woman was just lying to get him in trouble.

The sergeant told the man that he was in luck. He said that his department was quite fortunate because they had an in-house laboratory and they could just "swab" John's fingers to check out the woman's story. If John had not put his fingers into the woman's vagina, they would check out okay and he would be released. All of a sudden John hung his head and confessed that he was just trying to find out if she had been unfaithful. According to the sergeant, "what you see is not necessarily what you get." Indeed, things are not always as they first appear.

IT TOOK TWO MURDERS TO PROMPT CHANGE

San Diego Deputy Attorney Conducts Case Reviews

The San Diego Police Department began to enhance training on self-defense in DV cases in late 1992. This training was not further enhanced until late 1995. Unfortunately, it took the shocking deaths of two teenage girls to prompt this further enhancement.

A 17 year old girl who had previously been pushed and strangled by her ex-boyfriend was stabbed to death by him in the summer of 1995. This choking incident had not been pursued by the police department because the victim had suffered no visible injuries. Later the same summer, a 16 year old girl was strangled to death and set on fire by her ex-boyfriend. These deaths prompted Deputy City Attorney Gael Strack, with the blessing of City Attorney Casey Gwinn, to conduct a study of 300 DV incidents that all involved strangulation (Hawley et al., 2001; McClane et al., 2001; Strack, n.d.; Strack et al., 2001). All of these strangulation cases had been submitted for misdemeanor prosecution to the San Diego City Attorney's Office. The cases were evaluated to determine the signs and symptoms of attempted strangulation that could be used to corroborate the victim's allegation of being choked for purposes of prosecution. Strack began searching for a physician who could assist in this effort, and she located Dr. George McClane of Sharps Grossmont Hospital in La Mesa, CA to assist. He proved invaluable in determining injury patterns due to strangulation and strengthened the results of Strack's efforts.

Overall results revealed that a lack of adequate training had caused police and prosecutors to overlook symptoms of strangulation or to rely too heavily on the visible signs of strangulation. Because most victims of strangulation had no visible injuries or their injuries were too minor to photograph, opportunities for higher level criminal prosecution were often missed (Strack et al., 2001).

From the cases outlined above, Strack and her colleagues found that 59% of the suspects were employed and working in the following fields: professional (9%), business (24%), self-employed (3%), laborer (46%), skilled laborer (8%), and military (18%). The average age of the suspect was 31.9 years. Most of the victims were women (99%). The four cases involving women defendants were female to male (2), female to female (1), and mother to child (1). The majority of the time, the victim and perpetrator where intimately connected in some manner: victim's husband (25%), live-in partner (37%), parent of her child or "co-parent" (26%), former partner such as a husband, boyfriend, or live-in (6%), or a current boyfriend (6%). The average length of these relationships was 4.3 years.

Strack and colleagues also found that more victims reported being "choked" by their partner's hands (97%) than with a ligature (3%). When victims described being choked by their partner's hands (manual strangulation), they indicated that the suspect used one hand, two hands, an arm, or a "choke hold." Some women stated that they were strangled on the ground, bed, or sofa while being straddled by the suspect. Some victims stated that they were strangled while pinned against a wall. In some cases, the women reported that they were lifted off the ground during the strangulation. Most of the police reports simply indicated that the suspect "choked" the victim, without providing any further detail as to the method of strangulation. When a ligature was used to strangle the victim (garroting), suspects used objects such as electrical cords, mops, belts, ropes, towels, turtleneck sweaters, bras, or bathing suit tops. In one case, the victim reported that her boyfriend put a plastic bag over her head and tried to suffocate her. In addition, children witnessed the strangulation in at least 41% of the cases, although it is believed this number was probably higher because of reluctance of the victim to report that a child was present or because of failure of the officer to record the presence of children.

Focusing on the visible signs of strangulation, the data from Strack and colleagues show that while police officers documented an allegation of strangulation in all of the cases, they reported no visible injuries in about 50% of the cases. The majority of visible injuries observed by police officers appeared to be minor in nature and included red marks to the neck (often three red marks), thumb-print bruising (in one case, bruising was photographed two days later that was not apparent immediately after the incident), fingerprint bruising (either fingertips or digital outline of finger marks), long red scratch marks, bruising under the chin, on the jaw-line, or behind the ear(s), tiny red spots on the neck or eyes, or dual bloody-red eyes. Focusing on the symptoms, the following information was reported by victims and documented in police reports: "pain only" (located in either the neck or throat; 18%), voice changes (1%), breathing changes (5%), problems swallowing (2%), no symptoms documented or reported (67%), and other symptoms (7%). The other symptoms varied, including raspy voice, coughing, a sore throat, a sore throat for a few days, "throat felt like it closed down," nausea, vomiting, vomiting blood, pain to the ear, headaches, loss of consciousness, feeling like she was going to pass out, lightheadedness, seeing "black and white" or "black spots," hyperventilation, defecation, uncontrollable shaking, pupils not the same size, trouble walking, trouble moving neck, and loss of memory.

Strack and colleagues reported that when injuries were visible (149 cases), officers either took instant print photographs (114 cases) or did not take photographs because the injuries were described as "too minor to photograph" (35 cases). Of the 114 cases with photographs, only 45 cases contained photographs where an injury was visible in the picture (40%). There were 69 cases with unusable photographs (60%), either because the injuries were too minor to show up on a photograph or the photograph was of poor quality. Out of the total sample of 300 cases, only 15% (45 cases) had a photograph of sufficient quality to be used in court as physical evidence of strangulation. In other words, most victims of strangulation lacked sufficient physical evidence of being strangled because they either had no visible injury (50%) or their injuries were not photographed adequately (35%).

According to Strack and her colleagues, victims sought medical attention within 48 hours of the incident in only 5% of the cases. Medical attention appears to have been sought primarily because of persistent pain, voice changes, problems breathing, or trouble swallowing. When medical treatment was obtained, the medical observations were strikingly more robust. For example, in one case the officer described the visible injury as "red abrasion to the neck" while the attending physician described the same injury as "multiple linear contusions to both sides of neck with overlying redness, mild edema, and tenderness." The difference between the officer's description and the emergency physician's description is quite significant for a prosecutor.

Threats were documented in 40 cases, but specific threats were recorded by police in only a handful of cases (Table 1). A total of 10 victims identified themselves as being pregnant at the time of the incident. In one case, the victim had a miscarriage within 24 hours of being strangled. Interestingly, there was a history of prior DV in 89% of the cases that Strack and colleagues examined. In some of these cases, the suspect had been repeatedly prosecuted for DV by the City Attorney's Office, either with the same victim or a different victim, similar to findings elsewhere (Muelleman & Burgess, 1998; Wilson, 1977). These repeat offenders were likely to also have a criminal history involving other crimes, and a few were identified as gang members.

Overall, Strack and her colleagues found that 75% of the cases submitted for prosecution were either prosecuted as a new complaint or used for probation revocation. Prosecution of strangulation cases generally occurred only when there was enough evidence of injuries from other forms of violence, independent corroboration of being strangled, and/or a prior history of DV. Cases were rejected for prosecution (25%) when there was little corroboration of the strangulation or uncertainty regarding the identity of the primary aggressor due to failure in investigative procedures.

The finding that many suspects had a prior criminal history suggests that victims represented in Strack's results had experienced repeated violence over a significant period of time, and that the violence had escalated to the point of attempted strangulation–a felony and a potentially lethal level of violence. Given that most victims were also still living with the suspect in ongoing relationships with children present, they were at high risk for future violence.

Given the results of Strack's investigations, procedural changes were made. The procedural steps found in Table 2 are now included in a DV Unit officer's investigation and subsequent report. These procedures represent a major departure from the unspecified expectations under which many of the officers were previously operating.

TABLE 1. Specific Threats Used by Suspects During Strangulation of their Victims

Suspect Description	Verbalized Threat
Employed 42 year old male physician	"I can easily cut off your air supply by shutting off your carotid artery."
Employed 26 year old military male	"Dear God, please forgive me for what I am about to do."
Employed 33 year old laborer	"I'm going to choke you to death."
Unemployed 19 year old male	"I'm going to pop your neck."
Employed 26 year old military male	"I am going to commit an O.J. on you and leave no marks."
Employed 34 year old businessman	"Die, die."

SUMMARY AND CONCLUSIONS

As stated earlier, U.S. law enforcement agencies are typically paramilitary and patriarchal in organization and predominantly staffed by male officers. Given that victims of DV are overwhelmingly female, it is not hard to understand that male officers may often have little understanding of DV from a victim's perspective. Additionally, some officers may be unwilling to embrace the "new and progressive response" to DV, especially if it challenges personal stereotypical gender role beliefs. Some officers also tend to view all DV in terms of their own experiences in intimate relationships. It should be noted, however, that there are also many empathetic and very professional officers who provide wonderful service to victims. Many well-intentioned officers are simply not trained properly concerning DV in general, or in defensive injuries and strangulation in particular.

For these reasons, agencies should have specific, detailed policies and procedures regarding police response to DV incidents. However, it is important that these policies and procedures be more than just words on paper. Supervisors and other administrative personnel within the agency must monitor officer compliance. When officers fail to follow policies and procedures, either retraining or discipline must be imposed. My experience indicates that many agencies have wonderfully written policies, but they do not require compliance either through lack of officer monitoring/sanctioning or lack of priority in supervisor/administrative belief and action. In other words, clear investment in these policies and procedures must come from the top of the law enforcement hierarchy, or they will fail.

Training must be appropriate, broad, thorough, and comprehensive in the academy for new police officers, as well as during in-service training

TABLE 2. Procedural Steps at a DV Scene

ARRIVAL AT THE SCENE

1. Determine location and condition of victim.

2. Determine if suspect is still at scene.

3. Determine if any weapon is involved.

4. Determine what, if any, crime has occurred.

5. Summon ambulance if injuries require.

6. Separate the victim, suspect, and witnesses.

7. Prevent communication between the parties.

- This includes removing victim and witnesses from suspect's line of sight and range of hearing.

PRELIMINARY INVESTIGATION

1. Determine primary aggressor (primary aggressor is the person determined to be the most significant rather than the first aggressor). In identifying the primary aggressor, the officer shall consider:

    a. The intent of the law to protect victims of DV from continuing abuse;

    b. The threats creating fear of physical injury;

    c. The history of DV between the persons involved;

    d. Whether either person acted in self-defense.

2. Interview victim and witnesses separately, including any children who may have witnessed the incident or any prior incidents. *Do not* ask the victim whether he/she wishes to press charges.

    a. VICTIM: Note and document the following:

        i. Note the victim's physical condition, including:

            (a) Any injuries--describe in detail and determine if medical treatment is necessary and seek appropriate care;

            (b) Note torn clothing;

            (c) Note smeared makeup.

        ii. Note the victim's emotional condition.

        iii. Document any evidence of substance/chemical abuse by victim.

        iv. Determine victim's relationship to suspect.

        v. Conduct a lethality assessment by considering the following factors:

            ○ Is there a history of abuse?

            ○ Does the suspect have obsessive or possessive thoughts?

            ○ Has the suspect threatened to kill the victim?

            ○ Does the suspect feel he has been betrayed by the victim?

            ○ Is the victim attempting to separate from the suspect?

            ○ Have there been prior calls to the police?

            ○ Is there increasing drug or alcohol use by the suspect?

        ○   What is the prior criminal history of the suspect?

        ○   Is the suspect depressed?

        ○   Does the suspect have specific "fantasies" of homicide or suicide?

        ○   Does the suspect have access to or a fascination with weapons?

        ○   Has the suspect abused animals/pets?

        ○   Has the suspect demonstrated rage or hostile behavior toward police or others?

        ○   Has there been an increase in the frequency or severity of the abuse? (documented or not)

        ○   Has the suspect been violent toward children?

vi. Record any spontaneous statements of the victim.

vii. Obtain emergency contacts, telephone numbers, and pager numbers for the victim.

viii. Determine if there was strangulation involved and ask the questions contained in the Lethality Assessment (strangulation cases should be evaluated as *felony incidents*).

ix. Note any statements made by suspect to victim during incident.

b. WITNESSES: Note and document the following:

i. Interview all witnesses separately and record names, addresses, phone numbers and emergency contacts.

ii. List the names and ages of children present.

iii. Interview all children pursuant to protocol.

iv. Record names and addresses of emergency responder personnel.

v. Interview neighbors (including "ear-witnesses").

vi. Determine from witnesses if they are aware of a history of abuse.

c. SUSPECT: Note and document the following:

i. Describe suspect's location on arrival.

ii. Describe suspect's physical condition.

iii. Describe suspect's emotional condition.

iv. Document evidence of substance/chemical abuse by suspect, conduct examination, and add charge if appropriate.

v. Record spontaneous statements.

vi. Document, describe, and photograph any injuries.

vii. Admonish suspect and obtain waiver.

viii. Interview suspect.

d. EVIDENCE: Note and document the following:

i. Describe crime scene and note signs indicating struggle such as overturned furniture, hair that has been pulled out, blood, broken fingernails, holes in walls, damaged telephones, etc.

ii. Photograph crime scene if applicable.

iii. Determine if firearms or other deadly weapons are present and seize.

---

    iv. Ensure that victim's and suspect's injuries are photographed clearly.

    v. Impound and photograph all weapons and other evidence including all instrumentalities of the crime (i.e. belts, phone cords, hangers, gas cans, lighters, broken lamps, etc.).

    vi. In cases involving sexual assault, seize and appropriately impound clothing, bedding, or any material upon which the assault took place.

  e. MEDICAL TREATMENT: Note and document the following (if medical treatment is necessary):

    i. Transport or have victim transported to hospital.

    ii. Obtain names, addresses, and telephone numbers of ambulance or paramedic personnel treating the victim.

    iii. Document complaints of pain and injuries.

    iv. Obtain signed medical release from victim.

    v. Obtain copy of medical treatment form including doctor's name, address, and telephone number.

    vi. Interview treating physician and confirm nature and severity of injuries.

    vii. Determine if victim made statements to treating personnel regarding injury, incident or prior abuse.

    viii. Document all information.

COMPLETE THE CRIME REPORT

---

1. Maintain objectivity in reporting and avoid personal opinions regarding comments from victim/suspect.

2. Ensure that elements of all involved crimes are included in report.

3. Document any injuries victim has sustained on DV Supplemental form.

4. Make sure the victim was photographed.

    a. If a Polaroid camera was used, make sure the photographs clearly depict the injury or any object photographed.

    b. Photograph all children present, and the crime scene, if appropriate.

5. Document all evidence collected.

6. Document, in detail, any past history of physical violence. Describe the nature of the violence and whether it was reported or unreported.

* Adapted from San Diego Police Department's (1998) *Domestic Violence Law Enforcement Protocol.*

for tenured officers and front-line supervisors. The training should also incorporate issues such as male entitlement and bias, and not avoid or downplay these "hot button" topics. Finally, training must be updated and administered on a yearly basis in order to keep current with recent issues and findings, as well as reinforce the importance of DV policies and procedures within the ranks. If recommendations are implemented, it is expected that the rate of illegal victim arrests will be reduced.

REFERENCES

Breci, M. G. (2002). Police response to domestic violence. In J. E. Hendricks & B. D. Byers (Eds.), *Crisis intervention in criminal justice/social service* (pp. 119-140). Springfield, IL: Charles C. Thomas, Ltd.

Erez, E. (2002). Domestic violence and the criminal justice system: An overview. *Online Journal of Issues in Nursing, 7,* Manuscript 3. Retrieved August 19, 2002 from, http://www.nursingworld.org/ojin/topic17/tpc17_3.htm

Funk, M., & Schuppel, J. (2003). Strangulation injuries. *Wisconsin Medical Journal, 102,* 41-45.

Hamberger, L. K. (1997). Female offenders in domestic violence: A look at actions in context. *Journal of Aggression, Maltreatment, and Trauma, 1,* 117-129.

Hawley, D. A., McClane, G. E., & Strack, G. B. (2001). A review of attempted strangulation cases Part III: Injuries in fatal cases. *Journal of Emergency Medicine, 21,* 317-322.

Henning, K. Renauer, B. & Holdford, R. (2006). Victim or offender? Heterogeneity among women arrested for intimate partner violence. *Journal of Family Violence, 21*(6), 351-368.

Klein, A. R. (2004). *The criminal justice response to domestic violence.* Belmont, CA: Wadsworth Group.

Malloy, K. A., McCloskey, K. A., Grigsby, N., & Gardner, D. (2003). Women's use of violence within intimate relationships. *Journal of Aggression, Maltreatment & Trauma, 6,* 37-59.

McClane, G. E., Strack, G. B., & Hawley, D. A. (2001). A review of attempted strangulation cases Part II: Clinical evaluation of the surviving victim. *Journal of Emergency Medicine, 21,* 311-315.

Melton, H. C. (1999). Police response to domestic violence. *Journal of Offender Rehabilitation, 29,* 1-21.

Miller, S. L. (2001). The paradox of women arrested for domestic violence: Criminal justice professionals and service providers respond. *Violence Against Women, 7,* 1339-1376.

Mosher. D. L., & Sirkin, M. (1984). Measuring a macho personality constellation. *Journal of Research in Personality, 18,* 150-163.

Mosher, D. L., & Tomkins, S. S. (1988). Scripting the macho man: Hypermasculine socialization and enculturation. *Journal of Sex Research, 25,* 60-84.

Muelleman, R. L., & Burgess, P. (1998). Male victims of domestic violence and their history of perpetrating violence. *Academic Emergency Medicine, 6,* 866-870.

Murnen, S., Wright, C., & Kaluzny, G. (2002). If "boys will be boys," then will girls be victims? A meta-analytic review of the research that relates masculine ideology to sexual aggression. *Sex Roles, 46,* 359-583.

Pleck, E. (1987). *Domestic tyranny: The making of American social policy against family violence from Colonial times to the present.* New York: Oxford University Press.

Pretty, I. A., & Sweet, D. (2002). Anatomical location of bitemarks and associated findings in 101 cases from the United States. *Journal of Forensic Sciences, 45,* 812-4.

Robinson, A. L. (2000). The effect of a domestic violence policy change on police officers' schemata. *Criminal Justice and Behavior, 27,* 600-624.

Robinson, A. L., & Chandek, M. S. (2000). The domestic violence arrest decision: Examining demographic, attitudinal, and situational variables. *Crime & Delinquency, 46*(1), 18-37.

San Diego Police Department. (1998). *Domestic violence law enforcement protocol.* San Diego, CA: Author.

Smith, D. J., Mills, T., & Taliaferro, E. H. (2001). Frequency and relationship of reported symptomology in victims of intimate partner violence: The effect of multiple strangulation attacks. *Journal of Emergency Medicine, 21,* 232-329.

Stewart, A. (2001). Policing domestic violence: An overview of emerging issues. *Police Practice & Research, 2,* 447-459.

Stith, S. M. (1990). Police response to domestic violence: The influence of individual and familial factors. *Violence and Victims, 5,* 37-49.

Strack, G. B. (n.d). *"She hit me too:" Identifying the primary aggressor–a prosecutor's perspective.* San Diego, CA: San Diego City Attorney's Office. Retrieved August 16, 2004 from, http://www.ncdsv.org/images/She_hit_me.pdf

Strack, G. B., McClane, G. E., & Hawley, D. A. (2001). A review of attempted strangulation cases Part I: Criminal legal issues. *Journal of Emergency Medicine, 21,* 303-309.

Wilbur, L., Higley, M., Hatfield, J., Surprenant, Z., Taliaferro, E., Smith, D. J., et al. (2001). Survey results of women who have been strangled while in an abusive relationship. *Journal of Emergency Medicine, 21,* 297-302.

Wilson, J. Q. (1977). *Domestic violence and the police: Studies in Detroit and Kansas City.* Washington, DC: Police Foundation.

Worden, P. A. (2000). The changing boundaries of the criminal justice system: Redefining the problem and response in domestic violence. In C. M. Friel (Ed.), *Criminal justice 2000: Boundary changes in criminal justice organizations* (Vol 2., pp. 215-266). Washington, DC: National Institute of Justice.

Zorza, J. (1992). The criminal law of misdemeanor domestic violence, 1970-1990. *Journal of Criminal Law and Criminology, 83,* 46-72.

Submitted: October 1, 2004
Revised: January 19, 2007
Revised: May 3, 2007
Accepted: May 26, 2007

Victim-Defendants in Mandated Treatment: An Ethical Quandary

Donna Gardner

I have been providing services to battered women arrested for violent behavior against their abusers for the past nine years. I co-facilitate a group called "Women Who Resort to Violence" (WWRTV) with another facilitator from a local batterer intervention program. The group is held at the Artemis Center for Alternatives to Domestic Violence, an advocacy center in Dayton, OH that has been in operation for over 20 years.

It should be noted that the context for beginning and continuing this group has included the recent passage of a preferred arrest statute that often appears to be implemented as if it were a mandatory arrest statute, and a state that has no batterer intervention standards other than a voluntary set of standards endorsed by the Ohio Domestic Violence Network (ODVN). In the Dayton area alone, there are at least seven batterer intervention programs with very different requirements and philosophical foundations. For example, some programs accept both men and women into the same treatment groups, some focus on "anger issues" rather than on power and control dynamics, few are monitored by victim service agencies, and most give little recognition to the over-riding context or motivation for violence when assessing the individuals referred to them. Therefore, even while advocates have continued to educate members of the criminal justice system, it is apparent that victim defendants are still being mandated to intervention programs whether or not that particular program meets the ODVN standards. Within this context, the present article documents my experiences with women in the WWRTV group.

After spending two hours every Tuesday night for nine years working directly with battered women who have used violence or been accused of such, I have certainly been transformed by some of the strong feelings they bring to group. These feelings include anger, betrayal, grief, sorrow, frustration–specifically frustration with the criminal justice system and the domestic violence movement, both of which were supposed to be composed of people who would understand and provide a safety net for survivors using a wide range of strategies, including forms of social and legal resistance, to maintain safety.

Yet as advocates try to figure out how to best assist battered women caught up in the criminal justice system, we once again seem to be leaning toward a one-size-fits-all remedy such as the approach that got us into the situation in the first place (i.e., abused women being arrested for intimate partner violence [IPV] after poor implementation of preferred/mandatory arrest policies). Agencies that serve survivors of IPV are clamoring for some sort of alternative group curriculum or some other type of service for survivors who have been charged and convicted of IPV–related crimes. While many of us have the intention of treating each survivor as a unique person, there is still the tendency to find the quick fix–that is, to find some way to get around courts referring victims to batterer intervention and to reach out to those survivors who never planned to go to a victim-assistance agency, let alone be charged with IPV-related crimes.

Indeed, we should be doing all we can to right such injustices. But to what extent do those of us in the domestic violence movement re-victimize survivors by offering court-mandated groups such as WWRTV? Are we inadvertently legitimizing a miscarriage of justice? Are we simply perpetuating sorrow and further alienating women who might eventually want our services by implicitly agreeing with the label of 'perpetrator?' Might any survivor benefit from a mandated group? And whose voices do we listen to when making such decisions about offering services that the courts mandate? Regarding the last question posed, we obviously need to listen to the voices of victim-defendants themselves. However, we know this group is heterogeneous, with some who report that their lives are better and safer after having attended mandated treatment, while others report their lives are no better, and perhaps more complicated, as a result of being considered "bad enough" to warrant a sentence and subsequent referral. Thus, this article will offer far more questions than answers. Deep philosophical and practical issues abound when discussing best practices for survivors identified as battered women who are victim-defendants.

WOMEN'S USE OF VIOLENCE

Increased Arrests of Women:
Changes in the Law and Unintended Negative Consequences

In 1994, the state of Ohio passed legislation concerning domestic violence that was celebrated state-wide. The new law stated that arrest would be the preferred course of action for police officers called to an IPV incident. If officers did not make an arrest, documentation was required explaining why an arrest did not occur. After this law was passed, for various reasons many police agencies, on their own, instituted mandatory (rather than preferred) arrest policies for domestic violence calls.

Following these policy changes, more and more women were arrested for IPV within Ohio communities served by Artemis advocates. Women tended to plead guilty as charged, or plead guilty to a lesser charge. Reasons for these pleas varied as reported by women in the WWRTV group. Some women stated that they had children who needed them at home and could not afford to stay in jail any longer than they already had. Other women believed that since they had actually struck, slapped, and/or used other forms of violence found in police reports, they would be found guilty anyway. They sought to exit the system as quickly as possible–a system that did not understand them in the first place. Still other women reported that they never envisioned they would experience consequences such as probation, mandated treatment, or a criminal record that could haunt them for the rest of their lives. Interestingly, several survivors noted they had partners who had previously been processed through the courts and had not received any significant consequences for IPV (other than a criminal record that did not seem to affect their ability to work). Not surprisingly, many victim-defendants looked to the past criminal justice system experiences of their abusive partners as a predictor of what would happen to them. They were often quite wrong in their assumptions.

Rarely have women gone to trial for domestic violence in the jurisdictions that Artemis serves. This trend continues, and is one of the primary reasons that WWRTV groups have seen a major increase in women referred for treatment. This is similar to other locations in the U.S, where an increase in single or dual arrests of women has been documented (Crager, Cousin, & Hardy, 2003; Henning & Feder, 2004; Henning, Renauer, & Holdford, 2006; Klein, 2004; Martin, 1997; Miller, 2001). Over a decade ago, Hamberger and Potente (1994) first documented a large increase in women referred for batterer treatment following the implementation of mandatory and/or preferred IPV arrest policies in their communities. Hamberger and Guse (2002) also noted that while many different communities now dealt with increased arrests of battered women, no clear solutions to the problem had emerged.

Although many legal statutes require police at the scene to determine the primary batterer and then make arrests accordingly (Zamora, 2004), these statutes are often not being followed by police at the scene (O'Dell, this issue). Furthermore, Dasgupta (2002) outlined many of the moral and ethical concerns surrounding the arrest of women who have used violence in response to their own battering. She stated that "even the popular emerging rhetoric has marked women thus arrested as 'woman batterers'" (p. 1366). She goes on to say that identifying these women as batterers and "resocializing them to be nonviolent through education classes that are similar to men's programs seems illogical and inappropriate" (p. 1368). Thus, in this instance as an advocacy strategy, using the legal system as a means of protecting battered women has turned out to be much more complicated than previously supposed (DeLeon-Granados, Wells, & Binsbacher, 2006), and has created unintended and highly negative consequences for many abused women (McMahon & Pence, 2003).

Victims arrested for IPV may lose the ability to be self-sufficient through many pathways. Worcester (2002) states that having a criminal record often negatively affects career opportunities, child custody issues, immigration status, housing options, and the availability of social safety net funds such as Section VIII housing vouchers and welfare benefits. Bible and Osthoff (1998) also note that many of the careers heavily affected by having a criminal record are "...'women's work,' such as child care and health care jobs" (p. 8). These authors also state that a criminal record especially discriminates against women and their children precisely because "...as primary caretakers for their children, [they] are the ones [most likely] to apply for public benefits and housing" (p. 8). Renzetti (1999) states these issues are examples of widespread and common gendered injustice within our society.

Identifying the Primary Perpetrator of IPV

Worcester (2002) believes that "issues of power and control and the context of violence should be the foundation of policies and services regarding IVP and battered women's use of force" (p. 1391) in order to identify the primary batterer. For the criminal justice system, this would require an approach that runs counter to the prevailing lens of isolated and discrete incidents by including historical and contextual information, resulting in the need to almost completely overhaul the system itself. Indeed, McMahon and Pence (2003) remind us that "advocating for women in a sexist society is a radical act that cannot fit easily or comfortably in dominant institutions" (p. 49). Nevertheless, victims will continue to be arrested if police officers, prosecutors, and judges are not educated about the gendered nature of the factors that help identify primary batterers (Crager et al., 2003). Obvious and costly injustices will result from the failure to determine whether violence is part of a pattern of control, intimidation, and coercion (Dagsputa, 2002; Strauchler et al., 2004), or if it is a response within the context of self-defense and fear (Perilla, Frndak, Lillard, & East, 2003).

It should be noted that this is not a discussion about how frequently women or men are victimized. It is also not an attempt to provide the final word about women who have been victimized and are actively resisting. Instead, the discussion presented here focuses on the uniquely gendered expressions of women's IPV as it relates to determining the primary batterer. Worcester (2002) notes that it is important not to overlook the social, historical, and economic context of an individual's life when discussing the use of violence, especially the impact of multiple intersecting inequalities and gender roles. Society continues to fail many battered women of color, as well as battered women who are poor, drug or alcohol using, mentally ill, or from marginalized communities (Richie, 1995). Richie states:

> The choices are harder and the consequences are more serious for women with low incomes, women of color, lesbians, women who become pregnant at a young age, and others whose decisions, circumstance, and status violate the dominant culture's expectations....those whose lives are complicated by drug use, prostitution, undocumented immigrant status, low literacy, and a criminal record continue to be misunderstood, underserved, and isolated. (p. 11-12)

In addition to these types of inequalities, there are also gendered expectations for battered women. For example, women are not expected to react to their own victimization with violent resistance if they are to maintain the façade of being a "good woman" (McMahon & Pence, 2003; West, this issue). Thus, in the face of multiple constraints, women are expected to rationally, and in an orderly fashion, escape their abusers. The reality of multiple gendered barriers to this rational and orderly retreat (see Davis, this issue; Grigsby & Hartman, 1997) does not overcome the plaintive cry of "why doesn't she just leave?" still found emanating from many quarters (Anderson et al., 2003). Conversely, if a woman responds to her own victimization with violence, she is now increasingly likely to be arrested and thus revictimized by the justice system. Inconsistent and contradictory "double-bind" expectations are common for battered women, and constitute a major barrier to accurately identifying the primary batterer.

Despite this gendered double-bind, women continue to resist their own abuse in multiple ways (Goodman, Dutton, Weinfurt, & Cook, 2003). Some women utilize more socially accepted means such as calling the police, telling friends and family about the abuse, and learning about resources for battered women in their community. Other women engage in retaliation such as hiding their abusive partners' alcohol or cigarettes. Some intentionally resist their batterer's demands, such as actively seeking work and money independently of their abusive partner's wishes. Women also report utilizing internal resistance in the form of positive self-talk, thinking about what they would like to say in response to their abusers, and making plans for future change.

However, the rhetoric of zero tolerance found in such writings as Straus (1999, 2005) serves to decontexualize and equalize all violent acts between intimate partners at the level of topographic similarity, virtually ignoring the context, intent, or consequences related to these acts. Thus, in the words of McMahon and Pence (2003), IPV should be interpreted with "conditional tolerance and contextual sensitivity" (p. 66) in order to accurately identify the primary batterer, and yet often is not. In other words, not all slaps are created equal (Murphy & O'Leary, 1994; Osthoff, 2002). However, the insistence on proving gender equality within the IPV arena is nothing new. The debate over the appropriate definition of IPV continues (e.g., Saltzman, 2000), and currently there is still no universally accepted definition. Indeed, evidence of this ongoing definitional controversy can be seen in the recent infusion of multiple research publications targeting women's use of IPV (Bible, Dasgupa, & Osthoff, 2002-2003; Buttell & Carney, 2006; Cook & Swan, 2006; Frieze & McHugh, 2005; Hamberger, 2005; McHugh & Frieze, 2005).

Nevertheless, the motivation, intent, and consequences of violence within intimate relationships are quite different for men and women, and also vary within the context of the multiple inequalities mentioned above (Malloy, McCloskey, Grigsby, & Gardner, 2003). For example, Perilla et al. (2003)

states that "...the more options and resources that a woman sees as available to her, the more alternatives she will see to the use of violence . . . the effectiveness of violence as a deterrent to further abuse and victimization serves as a powerful reinforcer to young women whom society has failed to protect, and responding to violence with violence can appear a logical choice...." (p. 38). Without alternatives, violence may be the only option for many battered women, especially when confronting the choice between dying at the hands of an abuser or continuing to live.

SUMMARY

Women are being increasingly arrested for IPV and ordered into treatment. Battered women have found that their abusive partners are effective in charming the police into believing they have not been violent. Many victims have also been taken to jail after their abusers are successful in convincing police officers they are the injured party. Thus, many primary batterers have now added yet another tool to their abusive tool box that allows them to maintain power and control over their partners. Many batterers have found they now have the justice system at their disposal, and are able to manipulate the system in a way that is more damaging to their victims than they could have ever hoped.

Primary batterers are often well aware of how de-contextualized the criminal justice process is. When a victim utilizes physical violence or threats in retaliation, the predominant aggressor often strategically knows that the police will arrest her. Even when no violence is used, in some jurisdictions it is well-known that whoever calls the police first is assumed to be the victim regardless of degree of evidence, past criminal record, or other factors.

When abused women get to court, they often have to make difficult decisions with little information and even less time. Between being more likely to quickly plead guilty and being seen as an anomaly that must be seriously dealt with by the court system (e.g., a violent woman who clearly falls outside the predominant stereotype of femininity), women are increasingly finding themselves ordered to treatment for violent acts they committed within the context of their own victimization. It should not be surprising, then, that abused women often find that court-ordered treatment ranges from unhelpful to re-victimizing.

THE WOMEN WHO RESORT TO VIOLENCE (WWRTV) GROUP

Perilla et al. (2003) suggest that women's use of IVP is at least partially a result of learning, opportunity, and choice. Women may have learned, both within their intimate relationships as well as in the communities in which they live, that violence may elicit respect, or at least fear and compliance, from others. Violence often works to get what one needs, at least in the short term. The opportunity to use violence may be created by an abusive partner becoming incapacitated by drugs or alcohol, or it may simply be due to the availability of a knife on the kitchen counter next to where the survivor is standing. Alternatively, the choice to use violence may be an either/or proposition, such as whether to use violence or likely suffer extensive injury. The choice may also be a decision based on knowledge that little else has lessened the violence in the past.

Motivations for Women's Violence

An example of how this theory applies comes from a group member who attended WWRTV. During much of her childhood, Shauna[1] had witnessed her father assault and control her mother. She had also seen her mother self-defend and retaliate. Over time, her father stopped his physical assaults, which Shauna directly attributed to her mother's counter-assaults. When Shauna became involved with her latest intimate partner who is abusive and controlling, she knew that violence had worked for her mother in lessening her father's assaults. Shauna also knew she needed to take action immediately rather than wait until she was so hurt or depressed that it would be more difficult to take action. Finally, she made a clear choice about using violence in response to any violence she suffered from her partner.

Certainly many, if not all, women who come to the WWRTV group have used some form of resistance against the controlling tactics of their partners (Goodman et al., 2003). They may have shoved, slapped, thrown items, or simply refused to do something their partners demanded they do. Below is an account given by a WWRTV group member about how she ended up in treatment.

Although Cheryl had been married to Jerry for 10 years and had endured even more years of put-downs, shoves, thrown dishes, phones ripped out of walls, and threats to her and her family, this was the first time she had called the police. In her opinion, the most recent incident was much worse than past ones. She reported that she had physically fought back this time because she was tired of the stress, pain, and tears, but most of all she was tired of her children witnessing Jerry's violent behavior. In Cheryl's own words:

> It wasn't supposed to happen this way. I was supposed to be able to call the police, they would understand all I'd been through, and they would talk to him [Jerry] and make him understand that he'd better stop his abuse or he'd go to jail next time. The police would give me some agencies to call for help and take me seriously. It wasn't that I wanted to hurt him. I love Jerry. I just wanted him to know I'd reached my limit. When Jerry came into the kitchen sneering about how I do nothing during the day while he works so hard, I tried to tell him all the chores I'd done. Then he came right up to me and spit in my face! I was so shocked, I just moved away from the stove toward the sink to wipe my face. He came at me and pulled my pony-tail, yelling "Bitch, are you listening to me?!" That was it. It was like I physically felt something snap. I picked up the knife on the counter just to show him that I'd had enough, but when I turned around fast he was right there beside me and I cut his arm. I couldn't believe it. After all he'd done to me and here I was holding a knife, his arm bleeding. All I could think was how to stop the bleeding and now I was as bad as him. I dropped the knife and looked for a dishtowel to put on his arm. But Jerry said in this low voice that I'd better get out or he'd kill me. He just looked at me with those cold eyes and I knew I'd better go. So I ran down to my sister's house and called 911 from there. When the police arrived at my sister's, I went out to tell them how Jerry had threatened to kill me and had been violent in the past. The police went down the street to talk with Jerry and told me to stay at my sister's house. When they came back, they said I was under arrest for stabbing Jerry. I know I shouldn't have been surprised, but I was. I couldn't believe that I had finally called the police and I was the one going to jail.

Another survivor in the WWRTV group, Jeri, is no longer surprised that no one, including the police, will help her avoid her partner's violence. She states:

> There's nothing more I can do. I call the police, I get arrested. I try to move, he finds me. I try to get a job, he finds out and calls the employer and tells lies about me. He follows me everywhere. He threatens to kill my family. At this point I don't even leave my room.

When she was arrested for using force, she felt backed into a corner and saw no way to escape her former partner. Her response is similar to many others who have been mandated to the WWRTV group by local probation offices or children services. For Jeri, the safety net of a coordinated community response has many holes in it–holes she has fallen through every time she tried to rely upon it. At this point, while she doubts her own ability to help herself, she has found through experience that there is no one else who truly will.

These are but three examples of what might precipitate a battered woman's use of violence against her abuser. Women who use instrumental violence often have the goal of stopping a partner's violence and abuse. Sometimes they also wish to seek retribution, or somehow make the batterer understand all he has put her through. For victims who use violence, they may fall into one of the following categories: (a) immediate self-defense, or violence used during an assault to protect self or children; (b) delayed self-defense, or violence used soon after an assault when the victim feels she is still in imminent danger; (c) retaliatory violence, or violence used when imminent danger is passed, but still with the goal of demonstrating power in order to get a partner's violence to stop; (d) hyper-vigilant violence, usually used by women who have been victims of trauma by multiple offenders across the lifespan, who perceive a new threat or likelihood of abuse in the current environment, and whose response is often disproportionate to the current situation to make sure they are "never again" a victim; and (e) anticipator/preemptive violence, also used by women abused by multiple offenders across the life span, who use violence before any signal of a new threat, and seek to establish themselves as off-limits to any possible offender, real or perceived.[2] Certainly, these categories noted above are not mutually exclusive, nor should they be used to pigeon-hole battered women. Nevertheless, assessing for this type of motivation behind women's violence may allow us to intervene in more appropriate ways, especially if women themselves can see their own experiences and choices within the descriptions outlined above.

The women whose violence falls within the first two categories above have clearly acted in self-defense (immediate or delayed). Nevertheless, the criminal justice system is often not responsive to self-defense reasoning when female violence is involved. The third type of violence, retaliatory, is in a "nether region" that often makes sense only from the perspective of battered women or other victimized individuals, and is an extremely hard sell in most court rooms. The last two types, hyper-vigilant and participatory/preemptive, are clearly not seen as acceptable reasons for violent behavior, regardless of gender. However, some women who end up in the criminal justice system have not used violence, not even in self-defense. Instead, they were dealing with savvy batterers who knew that if they said the right things, the police would arrest their victims, again proving the batterers' omnipotence. When women have not been violent at all but are nevertheless referred to treatment, providers need to consider doing intense advocacy within the criminal justice system, as well as question the need for treatment. A clear needs-assessment with the referred women is warranted in order to determine if victim advocacy and support is wanted.

ENHANCING KNOWLEDGE AND SKILLS
FOR WORKING WITH BATTERED WOMEN
WHO USE VIOLENCE

An either/or perception of IPV has closed the doors of hope and safety to more than a few victims who have either used violence or otherwise become involved with the criminal justice system. In the not-so-good old days, one simply assumed that any woman who called a domestic violence crisis line must be a victim. If that victim were to say that she had been convicted of domestic violence, then there was a quick assumption that she was not someone who could be served with support, advocacy, or the other services that shelters and victim advocates provide. She would either be provided a referral to batterer intervention, a mental health provider, or simply denied services. Today that assumption is no longer valid. Victim service agencies are now recognizing the need to conduct full assessments for anyone calling a crisis line in order to both determine the primary batterer and to refrain from turning away those who could benefit and qualify for services.

In the case of Artemis, the agency that houses the WWRTV group, as we began completing more in-depth assessments of those victim-defendants who contacted us for mandated services, the muddier the waters became. Questions arose concerning how we should handle service provision, and certainly if we should provide any mandated services at all. This should continue to be a central question for any agency when discussing provision of a WWRTV group.

There are disturbing consequences to providing WWRTV-type groups. These consequences include but are not limited to: (a) arrested/convicted survivors may be mandated into treatment that runs counter to many of the core values of the advocacy field, such as self-determination and empowerment; (b) the criminal justice system may use such groups as an excuse to mandate victims into treatment, especially if victims are seen as more amenable to change compared to batterers; and (c) victim advocates may face the choice of whether or not to encourage prosecutors to mandate arrested victims into treatment as an alternative to conviction.

In fact, regarding this last point, McMahon and Pence (2003) encourage advocacy with prosecutors for reduced charges and WWRTV-type treatment in lieu of domestic violence convictions. This removes the extremely negative consequences of having an inaccurate domestic violence conviction on one's record. However, this approach clearly places both victims and victims' advocates in a double-bind when prosecutors present domestic violence conviction or mandated treatment as the only viable options.

Principles Based on the "Double-Bind": WWRTV-Type Groups

The WWRTV group, presented here as an advocacy-based template, was designed with the above double-bind in mind. The group curriculum was designed for IPV victims who have used violence against a partner in self-defense or retaliation (Waller, Malloy, & Gardner, 2002). Techniques and core values of the group are founded upon feminist theory, social learning theory, and cognitive behavioral theory. The goals are to empower the individual, increase knowledge, teach skills, and change attitudes through various methods including lecture, discussion, exercises, videos, and homework. Topics covered in group sessions include basic information about IPV dynamics and statistics, safety assessment and planning, anger management, healthy communication techniques, effects of IPV on parenting and children, and other key topics that allow for deeper reflection of the abuse that group members have endured, as well as survival skills they have developed (Waller et al., 2002).

One key method that is used in assessing the benefits and consequences of providing a WWRTV-type group for victim-defendants is talking directly with the women involved. Throughout their participation and at post-treatment, we ask the women about barriers that the treatment may have created, as well as opportunities. However, results are mixed. We have had women tell us that they believe group may have saved their lives. While they wish they would never have been arrested, convicted, or sentenced, they also believe they have better safety plans, are making better decisions for themselves, and more clearly understand IPV dynamics. They also often report a sense of relief from knowing that other women have experienced similar victimization and have similar feelings.

Conversely, other women participating in the WWRTV group have experienced great difficulties in securing transportation, getting time off from work, and/or securing childcare in order to attend treatment. Some also report that moving out of state and away from their batterers has been delayed as a result of probation requirements that dictate they must successfully complete the WWRTV in order to be released from mandated oversight. Thus, the very barriers that we as victim advocates must aid victims in overcoming (Grigsby & Hartman, 1997) can be the very ones we create for the women we serve unless we proceed with flexibility and responsiveness guided by victim safety, including intense advocacy with probation officers and judges.

Pairing WWRTV-Type Treatment with Creative Advocacy Strategies

It seems clear that advocates must seriously consider multiple strategies for overcoming such contradictions. McMahon and Pence (2003) offer categories concerning advocacy strategies on behalf of victims who resort to violence that encompass the criminal justice system from initial contact at the IPV scene to possible post-conviction sentencing and probation monitoring (see Table 1 for an expansion of these categories). These suggestions deal with the overall working of the system, but can also be tailored for use with an individual victim-defendant.

McMahon and Pence (2003) offer an important point–the single most effective remediation strategy concerning this problem would be to reduce the overall number of dual arrests within a jurisdiction. While this most certainly is important, some communities have found that a reduction in dual arrests still does not significantly reduce the number of battered women charged (Crager et al., 2003). A common statement heard from WWRTV group members during their first session is that the police told them "we have to arrest someone," with little primary batterer assessment conducted at the scene.

Once a victim is arrested, advocates should strongly consider intervening with both defense attorneys and prosecutors. Discussion with defense attorneys regarding the consequences of a trial versus pleading guilty should be considered, as well as educating defense attorneys about the long-term negative consequences of a conviction for victims. While working to change defense, prosecution, and sentencing strategies is certainly important, the fact remains that most women in the

TABLE 1. Advocacy for Victims Who Have Used Violence (adapted and liberally expanded from categories given in McMahon & Pence, 2003)

Police	Defense	Prosecutor	Sentencing/Rehab
- Review police reports where a woman is arrested for IPV.	- Work with defense attorneys to more aggressively defend women charged with assaulting their batterers.	- Educate prosecutors about the injustice of prosecuting victims acting in self-defense.	- Send only primary batterers to batterer treatment.
- Calculate those arrests of women that may have been self-defense.	- Educate defense lawyers about the long-term consequences to victims of pleading guilty.	- Work to increase understanding of the gendered nature of IPV.	- Send victims who have used violence to WWRTV-type groups.
- Train officers on determination of self-defense in IPV cases.		- Educate prosecutors about the risks to victims no longer willing to remain passive.	- Educate judges and probation officers about the differences in treatment needs.

WWRTV group say that the "worst part of the nightmare" was being arrested (often in front of their children), put in a police car, and then spending time in jail. Injustice and the shattering of faith in the criminal justice system occur long before the victim-defendant's case reaches a prosecutor.

CONCLUSIONS: CONFRONTING CRITICISM

It seems clear we should conduct aggressive advocacy to take up the cause of women who are victim-defendants. Victim advocates have an obligation to educate others and state the case appropriately. Explaining primary batterer assessment approaches more strenuously and in a detailed manner can only help. It is important that advocates inform defense attorneys, prosecutors, judges, and probation officers about the miscarriage of justice that occurs when primary batterer assessments are not appropriately completed, often resulting in the arrest and conviction of battered women.

Advocacy within the justice system about injustices it has committed against IPV victims certainly is not easy. It is difficult to introduce a change of focus within this system to create sensitivity to the patterns and contexts important to IPV. It is also difficult to overcome feelings of frustration and hopelessness held by many criminal justice professionals concerning the "revolving door" issue of repeat offenders and victims. In addition, advocates often face an uphill battle in overcoming the stereotypes that most advocates are man-haters who refuse to believe that men could ever be IPV victims (Klein, 2004).

Despite these often entrenched roadblocks to change, advocates must remain aware of the everyday and sometimes mundane forms of injustice that victim-defendants face. Every time women gather for the WWRTV group, there is always at least one victim who discusses the difficulty in simply showing up, ranging from problems with bus schedules to securing safe and adequate child care. Every group, there is always at least one victim who discusses her frustration that her abusive partner is not being held accountable for his violent behavior. All the while, we as facilitators must question whether or not we have created an easy rationalization used by the criminal justice system to justify the arrest and conviction of IPV victims.

Have we made it easier for the criminal justice system to arrest and convict IPV victims because now there is a mechanism to "reform" them? Quite possibly. Should we focus advocacy efforts on educating police, prosecutors, probation officers, and judges, as well as modifying existing laws, so it is not as easy to charge victims who self-defend, retaliate, or are not violent at all? Absolutely.

Should those of us who live in states in which there are no required batterer intervention standards advocate for them so that no victim is put in a group with primary batterers? Should we spend our time educating traditional batterer intervention providers and gaining consensus about service to victims who have used violence? Should we research and modify primary batterer assessment tools and then market them to members of the criminal justice system so that victims and batterers are correctly identified? Have we become co-opted by the very system we originally tried to reform? Does a treatment group for women who use violence or who, in some way, have become defendants in the criminal justice system and are mandated to attend, benefit them or empower them in any way? How, if at all, can an agency that prioritizes empowerment for victims provide a group that requires their attendance as a result of their methods of resisting the abuse they are experiencing? How can we, with limited resources, simultaneously address the needs of today's victim defendants while achieving system change?

These are but a few of the questions we must consider as we offer services to victim-defendants mandated to treatment. There is no best answer concerning how we should respond to the current situation of battered women arrested for IPV. Clearly traditional batterer intervention is not an answer. Yet also as clearly, we have yet to find the best answers for the victim-defendants now involved in a system that, even with our best advocacy efforts, may not recognize their unique needs for years.

NOTES

1. All names of victims and perpetrators are pseudonyms for reasons of confidentiality.

2. Certainly there are women who are primary aggressors whose coercive violence is used as a means to establish power and control over a partner, and not as a protective measure. Women who are primary aggressors are beyond the scope of this discussion.

REFERENCES

Anderson, M. A., Gillig, P. M., Sitaker, M., McCloskey, K., Malloy, K., & Grigsby, N. (2003). "Why doesn't she just leave?" A descriptive study of victim reported impediments to her safety. *Journal of Family Violence, 18*(3), 151-155.

Bible, A., Dasgupa, S., & Osthoff, S. (Eds.). (2002-2003). Women's use of violence in intimate relationships: Part 1, 2, 3 [Special issues]. *Violence Against Women, 8*(11-12), 9(1).

Bible A., & Osthoff, S. (1998). When battered women are charged with assault. *Double-Time: Newsletter of the National Clearinghouse for the Defense of Battered Women, 6*(1/2), 8-10.

Buttell, F. P., & Carney, M. M. (Eds.) (2006). *Women who perpetrate relationship violence: Moving beyond political correctness*. Binghamton, NY: Haworth Press.

Cook, S. L., & Swan, S. C. (Eds.) (2006). Special issue. *Violence Against Women, 12*(11).

Crager, M., Cousin, M., & Hardy, T. (2003). *Victim-defendants: An emerging challenge in responding to domestic violence in Seattle and the King County region*. St. Paul, MN: Minnesota Center Against Violence and Abuse (MINCAVA). Retrieved April 14, 2005 from, www.mincava.umn.edu/documents/victimdefendant/victimdefendant.pdf

Dasgupta, S. D. (2002). A framework for understanding women's use of nonlethal violence in intimate heterosexual relationships. *Violence Against Women, 8*(11), 1364-1389.

Davis, D. A. (2007). Non-violent survival strategies in the face of intimate partner violence and economic discrimination. *Journal of Aggression, Maltreatment & Trauma, 15*(3/4), 123-153.

DeLeon-Granados, W., Wells, W., & Binsbacher, R. (2006). Arresting developments: Trends in female arrests for domestic violence and proposed explanations. *Violence Against Women, 12*, 355-371.

Frieze, I. H., & McHugh, M. C. (Eds.) (2005). Special issue: Female violence against intimate partners. *Psychology of Women Quarterly, 29*(3).

Goodman, L. A., Dutton, M. A., Weinfurt, K., & Cook, S. (2003). The Intimate Partner Violence Strategies Index: Development and application. *Violence Against Women, 9*(2), 163-186.

Grigsby, N., & Hartman, B. R. (1997). The barriers model: An integrated strategy for intervention with battered women. *Psychotherapy, 34,* 485-498.

Hamberger, L. K. (Ed.) (2005). Special issue on men's and women's use of intimate partner violence. *Violence and Victims, 20*(3).

Hamberger, L. K., & Guse, C. E. (2002). Men's and women's use of intimate partner violence in clinical samples. *Violence Against Women, 8*(11), 1301-1331.

Hamberger, L. K., & Potente, T. (1994). Counseling heterosexual women arrested for domestic violence: Implications for theory and practice. *Violence and Victims, 92*(2), 125-137.

Henning, K., & Feder, L. (2004). A comparison of men and women arrested for domestic violence: Who presents the greater threat? *Journal of Family Violence, 19*(2), 69-80.

Henning, K., Renauer, B., & Holdford, R. (2006). Victim or offender? Heterogeneity among women arrested for intimate partner violence. *Journal of Family Violence, 21*(6), 351-368.

Klein, A. R. (2004). *The criminal justice response to domestic violence.* Belmont, CA: Wadsworth/Thompson.

Malloy, K. A., McCloskey, K. A., Grigsby, N., & Gardner, D. (2003). Women's use of violence within intimate relationships. *Journal of Aggression, Maltreatment & Trauma, 6*(2), 37-59.

Martin, M. (1997). Double your trouble: Dual arrest in family violence. *Journal of Family Violence, 12*(2), 139-157.

McHugh, M. C., & Frieze, I. H. (Eds.) (2005). Special issue: Understanding gender and intimate partner violence: Theoretical and empirical approaches. *Sex Roles, 52*(11-12).

McMahon, M., & Pence, E. (2003). Making social change: Reflections on individual and institutional advocacy with women arrested for domestic violence. *Violence Against Women, 9*(1), 47-74.

Miller, S. (2001). The paradox of women arrested for domestic violence: Criminal justice professionals and service providers respond. *Violence Against Women, 7*(12), 1-24.

Murphy, C. M., & O'Leary, K. D. (1994). Research paradigms, values, and spouse abuse. *Journal of Interpersonal Violence, 9*(2), 207-223.

O'Dell, A. (2007). Why do police arrest victims of domestic violence? The need for comprehensive training and investigative protocols. *Journal of Aggression, Maltreatment & Trauma, 15*(3/4), 53-73.

Osthoff, S. (2002). But Gertrude, I beg to differ, a hit is not a hit is not a hit: When battered women are arrested for assaulting their partners. *Violence Against Women, 8*(12), 1521-1544.

Perilla, J. L., Frndak, K., Lillard, D., & East, C. (2003). A working analysis of women's use of violence in the context of learning, opportunity, and choice. *Violence Against Women, 9*(1), 10-46.

Renzetti, C. (1999). The challenge to feminism posed by women's use of violence in intimate relationships. In S. Lamb (Ed.), *New visions of victims: Feminists struggle with the concept* (pp. 42-56). New York: New York University Press.

Richie, B. E. (1995). *Compelled to crime: The gender entrapment of battered black women.* New York: Routledge.

Saltzman, L. E. (2000). Guest Editor's introduction to the Special Issue: Building data systems for monitoring and responding to violence against women, part II. *Violence Against Women, 6*(8), 811-814.

Strauchler, R., McCloskey, K., Malloy, K., Sitaker, M., Grigsby, N., & Gillig, P. (2004). Humiliation, manipulation, and control: Evidence of centrality in domestic violence against an adult partner. *Journal of Family Violence, 19*(6), 339-354.

Straus, M. A. (1999). The controversy over domestic violence by women: A methodological, theoretical, and sociology of science analysis. In X. B. Arriage & S. Oskamp (Eds.), *Violence in intimate relationships* (pp. 17-44). Thousand Oaks, CA: Sage.

Straus, M. A. (2005). Women's violence toward men is a serious social problem. In D. R. Loseke, R. J. Gelles, & M. M. Cavanaugh (Eds.), *Current controversies on family violence* (2nd ed., pp. 55-77). Thousand Oaks, CA: Sage.

Waller, C., Malloy, K., & Gardner, D. (2002). *Group intervention curriculum for women who resort to violence.* Dayton, OH: Artemis Center for Alternatives to Domestic Violence and Wright State University School of Professional Psychology PATH Program.

West, C. M. (2007). "Sorry, we have to take you in:" Black battered women arrested for intimate partner violence. *Journal of Aggression, Maltreatment & Trauma, 15*(3/4), 95-121.

Worcester, N. (2002). Women's use of force: Complexities and challenges of taking the issue seriously. *Violence Against Women, 8*(11), 1390-1415.

Zamora, E. C. (2005). *Enhanced penalties for domestic violence 2005.* Retrieved May 1, 2007 from, http://data.ipharos.com/bwjp/documents/Enhanced%20Penalties%202005.pdf

Submitted: May 3, 2005
Revised: January 19, 2007
Revised: May 4, 2007
Accepted: May 26, 2007

"Sorry, We Have to Take You In:" Black Battered Women Arrested for Intimate Partner Violence

Carolyn M. West

Anti-violence activists, mental health service providers, shelter workers, and researchers recognize that women sometimes use violent tactics against their male intimate partners, yet many have been, and continue to be, reluctant to engage in candid discussions about this topic. The fear of jeopardizing funding and support for essential services for battered women, among other reasons, has discouraged a meaningful, respectful exchange about female-perpetrated intimate partner violence (IPV). However, more books (e.g., Buttell & Carney, 2006; Miller, 2005), special journal issues (e.g., Bible, Dasgupta, & Osthoff, 2002-2003), and workshops (Rosen, 2006) are currently being devoted to this complex, challenging, and controversial subject.

The literature on women's use of IPV has broadly reflected one of two themes. The first theme reflects a family violence gender symmetry perspective. Using community and nationally representative samples, family violence investigators discovered that similar rates of IPV perpetration were reported by women and men who were in dating, cohabitating, or marital relationships (Archer, 2000; Dutton, Nicholls, & Spidel, 2005). Moreover, whether reported by couples or in comparison samples of males and females, a significant number of respondents described mutual or bidirectional violence (Caetano, Ramisetty-Mikler, & Field, 2005). The second theme concerns a contextual analysis that illuminates gender differences in the context, motivation, results, and consequences of IPV. Contextual researchers have provided compelling evidence that men's and women's use of violence is seldom comparable or symmetrical, especially when clinical samples or agency data are used (e.g., courts, police agencies, hospitals, and shelters; Hamberger, 2005; Kimmel, 2002).

The tension between these two camps represents more than just an academic debate. The way in which women's use of IPV is framed by scholars and other stakeholders can trigger institutional responses by the criminal, legal, or mental health systems that can either be helpful or inadvertently revictimize the survivor. For example, some legal professionals, such as police officers and prosecutors, have asserted that the punishment for domestic violence should be gender neutral and that those women who use force against intimate partners "...should be arrested the same as a man. We should not differentiate just because she's a female" (Miller, 2001, p. 1353). However, there is a great deal of heterogeneity among women who are arrested for using IPV. A substantial number of female arrestees, 60% in some samples, are actually battered women who have used aggression in the context of ongoing abuse perpetrated against them by male partners (for a review, see Rajan & McCloskey, this issue). Criminalizing these women for physical resistance or self-defense obviously has serious consequences. For instance, victims arrested for IPV may well be reluctant to seek future assistance from the legal system, be denied access to shelters and protection orders, or even be court-ordered to attend batterer treatment programs (Henning, Renauer, & Holdford, 2006).

On the other hand, front-line service providers such as advocates and therapists contend that women often used violence in self-defense and should not be arrested along with, or instead of, primary male aggressors. Instead, these women should be categorized as "victim-defendants" (Crager, Cousin, & Hardy, 2003). Yet it is important to acknowledge that a small proportion of women arrested for IPV, approximately 1-7% across recent samples, appear to be primary aggressors (Rajan & McCloskey, this issue). Similar to their male counterparts, these primary female perpetrators should be held accountable by the legal system or enrolled in appropriate batterer treatment programs (Henning et al., 2006). How this debate is resolved, and whether or not victim-defendants who use violence should receive punishment, treatment, or some other form of intervention, will most likely have a disproportionate impact on the lives of Black women.

After decades of research, investigators have documented the presence of IPV across ethnic and socioeconomic groups. It has also been shown that the economic and social marginalization of Black women is associated with elevated rates of both IPV victimization and perpetration (Potter, 2006). As a result of the frequency and severity of violence in their lives, Black women have the propensity to use aggression to protect themselves and their children or in retaliation against intimate abusers. Consequently, a disproportionate number of Black women may be categorized as mutual combatants, or even primary aggressors, and later arrested. Paradoxically, legal reforms, such as mandatory arrest polices that were originally designed to protect victims, have been associated with an increased number of women, particularly Black women, being arrested for IPV (Melton & Belknap, 2003; Simpson, Bouffard, Garner, & Hickman, 2006).

Accordingly, the purpose of the present effort is to examine the experiences of Black victim-defendants. In the first section, I will present an integration of both the family violence gender symmetry perspective and the contextual perspective to review the literature on Black women's use of violence within heterosexual relationships, and introduce the concept of *bidirectional asymmetric violence* as a result of that integration. In the second section, I will explore possible factors that may contribute to Black women's overrepresentation in the legal system, including the enactment of mandatory arrest laws. Black feminist scholars have used life histories to document the experiences of Black victim-defendants to good effect (e.g., Richie, 1996). Similarly, the third section will describe the experiences of one Black female victim who was arrested after using physical aggression to defend herself against an abusive boyfriend. Finally, strategies for advocacy and intervention are offered.

BLACK WOMEN'S USE OF VIOLENCE

Bidirectional Asymmetric Violence

High rates of female-perpetrated dating violence have been documented among adolescent Black youth (West & Rose, 2000). For example, when compared to their male counterparts, Black female college students (35% vs. 47%, respectively) reported using more physical aggression within their dating relationships, such as pushing, slapping, and hitting (Clark, Beckett, Wells, & Dungee-Anderson, 1994). Cohabitating and married Black women have reported aggression against their boyfriends and husbands as well. According to the National Family Violence Surveys, the rate of Black husband battering increased from 76 per 1,000 in 1975 to 108 per 1,000 in 1985. Although this 42% increase in IPV was not statistically significant, this finding led some researchers to conclude that a growing number of Black men have experienced IPV victimization (Hampton, Gelles, & Harrop, 1989).

It should be noted, however, that a substantial number of couples are involved in mutual or bidirectional aggression. Among the violent Black couples in the National Alcohol Survey, the rate of self-reported bidirectional partner violence (61%) was two times that of unidirectional female-to-male partner violence (31%) and about six times higher than unidirectional male-to-female partner violence (8%). One-third of Black couples who reported bidirectional partner violence described it as severe, defined by such descriptors as beat up, choked, raped, or threatened with a weapon (Caetano et al., 2005). When the couples were re-interviewed five years later, 17% of the Black couples continued to engage in mutual violence (Field & Caetano, 2005). Interestingly, the occurrence of higher rates of bidirectional partner violence among Black couples, when compared to their White and Hispanic counterparts, was independent of education, income, employment status, alcohol problems, and history of violence in the family of origin. Researchers concluded that ". . . violence among Blacks is more likely to be mutual violence where both partners are committing and being exposed to partner violence" (Caetano et al., p. 401).

However, mutuality of violence does not mean that women's and men's violent acts are equal. While both partners may use violence, when taken in context it is evident that the frequency and severity of their assaults are seldom equal. These relationships may be better characterized as bidirectional asymmetric violence. The following scenario is offered to illustrate this point: A wife shoves and scratches her husband. He then punches her in the face and breaks her nose. In other words, although this scenario is an example of bidirectional IPV in that both partners are violent, the outcome is asymmetrical because the wife sustained the most serous injury (Temple, Weston, & Marshall, 2005).

Moreover, there are often significant gender differences in the types, frequency, and severity of aggressive acts committed by perpetrators. For example, Swan and Snow (2002) interviewed a predominately Black sample of 108 low-income women who had used physical violence against a male partner during the previous six months. The authors found that women and men committed equivalent levels of emotional and verbal abuse (e.g., yelling, screaming, name calling). Women also perpetrated significantly more moderate physical violence than their male partners, defined as throwing objects, pushing, and shoving. In contrast, women reported that their male partners engaged in significantly more severe acts of physical violence such as choking, sexual aggression, and coercive control. Male perpetrators were more prone to restrict their partners' use of the car, telephone, or access to family and friends, and to prevent their partner from leaving the house, seeking medical care, or obtaining employment. When Black women attempted to use coercive control, they used fewer controlling acts and were less successful in controlling their partner's behavior. The researchers concluded that "although these women were just as or more violent, the partners were still controlling the women's behavior" (p. 303).

Intersecting Oppressions

In addition, IPV obviously occurs within a social, historical, and economic context in which Black women are often disadvantaged. Alternatively stated, Black women's use of force and their reactions to abuse are affected by their social location and place in society. Living at the intersection of multiple forms of oppression, including but not limited to race, class, and gender discrimination, increases the probability that Black women will be economically disadvantaged and will experience IPV as both victims and perpetrators (Potter, 2006). For example, as with Black male-to-female violence, Black couples who reported female-to-male partner violence had significantly lower mean annual incomes (Cunradi, Caetano, & Schafer, 2002) and were more likely to live in impoverished neighborhoods (Cunradi, Caetano, Clark, & Schafer, 2000).

Several factors may account for the association among poverty, residence in economically disadvantaged neighborhoods, and Black female-perpetrated IPV. Low-income urban areas are often characterized by racial segregation, social isolation, rampant unemployment, and community violence, including high rates of non-IPV homicide. In these communities, the appearance of physical or emotional weakness can be dangerous, making at least the show of violence essential for survival. When violence is routinely modeled for Black women (and men) as a way of achieving one's goals, as a means of self-protection, or as a conflict resolution strategy, this aggressive behavior can easily spill over into intimate relationships (Benson & Fox, 2004; Websdale, 2001).

In order to cope with the stress and trauma of living in such harsh conditions, individuals may drink or use drugs, which is also associated with IPV. Alcohol-related problems are strongly related to both Black female and male perpetrated IPV (Cunradi, Caetano, Clark, & Schafer, 1999). With few economic resources to escape the violence, coupled with limited access to social services such as battered women's shelters, some impoverished women may resort to IPV homicide. For example, some researchers suggest that since welfare benefits have declined, more unmarried Black males have been killed by their girlfriends (Dugan, Nagin, & Rosenfeld, 2003). On the other hand, the most recent U.S. justice system data show that, for the year 2004, Black females killed by a spouse or ex-spouse were 2.76 per 100,000 population, compared to Black males (1.12 per 100,000), suggesting that Black females are still about 2.5 times more likely than Black males to be murdered by their marriage partners (Fox & Zawitz, 2006). Similarly for unmarried partners (girlfriend/boyfriend), Black females were about twice as likely to be killed by their intimates compared to Black males (3.49 and 1.75 per 100,000, respectively).

BLACK WOMEN AS VICTIM-DEFENDANTS

Beginning in the 1980s, legislative attention to the problem of IPV has led to the enactment of an avalanche of laws across the U.S. In fact, between 1997 and 2003, more than 700 laws were created, including both amendments to old laws and enactment of new laws. For example, many jurisdictions enacted mandatory arrest policies that required police officers to detain a person based on a probable cause determination that a domestic assault had occurred and that the accused person had indeed committed the offense. Pro-arrest laws considered arrest to be the preferred, but not the required action in domestic violence incidents. "No drop" policies also were established that required the prosecution of batterers, regardless of a victim's recantation or pleas for leniency. These laws were designed to send a clear message to the public that IPV is a serious crime that will not be tolerated, as well as to empower and protect victims and to prevent selective enforcement of laws based on extralegal factors such as race and social class (for reviews, see Miller, 2003, 2004).

Undoubtedly, legal interventions have saved the lives of many victims and their children. However, the enactment of mandatory/pro-arrest legislation has had several unintended negative consequences, including a measurable rise in the single and dual arrests of women in which victims are been arrested along with their abusers (DeLeon-Granados, Wells, & Binsbacher, 2006). Although this arrest pattern has occurred across ethnic groups, Black women are being arrested and incarcerated at higher rates. To illustrate, after pro-arrest legislation was expanded in Maryland, there was an increase in the number of White women being arrested, with 18% detained before and 25% after the new law was implemented. The increase was even more dramatic for Black women, with 25.3% and 38% being arrested before and after the policy, respectively (Simpson et al., 2006).

The severity of IPV assaults perpetrated by Black women may be one factor that explains these higher arrest rates. As evidence, using police records concerning a predominately Black sample, researchers have compared the demographic characteristics, criminal history, and the past IPV history of men and women who had been arrested. Compared to male defendants, more females bit, hit, scratched, threw an object, used a weapon, or struck their partner with a vehicle (Melton & Belknap, 2003). Although female arrestees were no more likely than their male counterparts to have injured their partner/spouse during the incident for which they had been arrested, more women had used a weapon during the incident, perhaps to level the playing field once abuse had begun. The use of deadly force may explain why more women had been charged with a felony assault (Henning & Feder, 2004).

However, there is compelling evidence that a substantial number of female arrestees are actually battered women who have been arrested after they used violence to defend themselves. In a sample of Black couples who were dually arrested, more male arrestees had choked, sexually assaulted, threatened, or actually used a weapon against their victim when compared to female arrestees (Feder & Henning, 2005). Equally as disturbing, more male arrestees had pushed, shoved, hit, or threatened a child during the attack or had made homicidal threats against themselves, the female arrestee, or the children if the victim attempted to end the relationship. In addition, more male arrestees had attacked their partner after a separation, had a gun in the house, and had violated existing protection orders (Feder & Henning). Understandably, female defendants reported greater fear and cited self-defense more often as the primary motivation for their aggressive acts (Melton & Belknap, 2003).

Taken together, the research indicates that an alarmingly high number of Black women have assaulted their male partners or have been involved in mutually abusive relationships (Caetano et al., 2005). However, Black women's use of violence often occurs in the context of gender inequality in which their aggression lacks the same meaning and impact as their male partner's violence. More specifically, Black women assaulted their partners, sometimes severely enough to cause in-juries, yet they also sustained injuries, experienced mental health prob-lems as a result of the abuse, and generally lacked the power to use coercive control to terrorize and subjugate their male partners (Swan & Snow, 2003).

While middle- and upper-middle class Black women may also be in-volved in IPV (Lockhart & White, 1989), poverty and residence in im-poverished communities can curtail the ability of many poor couples to create nurturing, nonviolent relationships. Consequently, economically disadvantaged Black women are at elevated risk for inflicting and sus-taining IPV (Cunradi et al., 2000, 2002). Paradoxically, enforcement of mandatory/pro-arrest laws that were intended to protect IPV victims has oftentimes resulted in unintended consequences. Indeed, more women, particularly Black women, have been arrested as a result. When the con-text of violent heterosexual relationships is considered, it appears that a substantial number of these women are arrested after using force to protect themselves (Melton & Belknap, 2003).

IRENE'S STORY

Black feminist scholars have used life histories and narratives to doc-ument the experience of battered Black women who have been arrested for IPV (e.g., Richie, 1996). Accordingly, I will describe the experi-ences of Irene (not her real name). Irene is a 41-year-old Black woman who has an extensive history of IPV as both a victim and perpetrator. I met her in 1997, shortly after I moved to Washington state. In 2001, Irene began dating Dennis, a 38-year-old Caucasian man, who quickly became controlling and violent. Several months later, Irene attempted to terminate the relationship. After she had used violence to defend her-self from a potentially lethal attack, she was arrested for assault and incarcerated for several days.

During Irene's relationship with Dennis, I frequently spoke with her about the abuse. Following her arrest, I also reviewed the court tran-scripts, attended her trial, and offered emotional support. After receiv-ing permission from the Human Subjects Review Board at my location, I conducted two tape-recorded interviews with Irene (each lasted more than two hours). My purpose was to use Irene's words to vividly capture the experience of one Black woman victim-defendant.

First, I describe below how she and Dennis met and present some early indicators of his abusive nature. I then follow this with a description of the most serious violent event that led to Irene's arrest. Next, I describe the arrest, her time in jail, and the trial. The section ends with a case analysis and discussion.

The Meeting and Relationship

Life was good for Irene. After many years of working for other shop owners, she had purchased her own beauty salon. Dennis walked into her salon in March of 2001. He was a 38-year-old White man with striking blue eyes, and his 295 pounds looked good on his 6'3" frame. Monday afternoons were slow, which left time to chat while she cut his hair. Irene was impressed because Dennis appeared to be the "complete package." He disclosed he was a single parent of a small son who had moved back home to care for an aging mother. He also said he worked as a professional pilot while balancing his family obligations. This suggested that he was intelligent, educated, and responsible. "Wow," Irene thought, "when a man said 'I'm raising my 3 year old son alone,' that automatically put him at a level of respectability and status." Her emotional involvement grew after she met Dennis' son, Howard. Irene felt that this adorable child and his father, who both appeared to be vulnerable, needed female attention. Although she did not have children of her own, she believed that her nurturing tendencies made her the perfect person for a new maternal role.

It was official: Irene was in love. She quickly became immersed in Dennis' life. He provided new adventures, including camping trips and flights in his private airplane. She even learned to appreciate country western music. The relationship went well for five or six months, although maintaining the relationship began to feel like a chore. Dennis made frequent calls to the salon, which disrupted Irene's work. After a long work day, Irene sometimes wanted a hot bath and a quiet evening alone. "It became like they were imposing on me," she said.

During December of 2001, a job opportunity took Dennis and Howard to Alaska. This was a good time for Irene to explore her feelings about the relationship. Although Irene was hopeful, family members and friends, myself included, thought the relationship was unhealthy and dangerous. More specifically, Dennis appeared to be marginally employed, yet he returned from several "business trips" with stacks of cash. I suggested that Irene inquire about the nature of these lucrative business ventures. In addition, Dennis exhibited signs of alcoholism. Although there were periods of sobriety, abstinence made him shake and tremble. When liquor was unavailable, he drank cough syrup or took pills to overcome these symptoms, and Irene found herself buying alcohol to temporarily help him feel better.

In addition, Dennis had an arsenal of weapons and a very bad temper, which he routinely displayed to Irene and others. In one particular instance, the neighborhood antiques dealer had offended Irene and her multiracial clientele by bringing a "Colored Only" sign into her salon. For them, this piece of "art" was a reminder of the painful days of segregation. When Irene described the upsetting racial incident to Dennis, he confronted the antiques dealer and threatened to "shove my gun up your tailbone if you bother my Black woman again!" In another instance, there was the July 4th camping trip. After nightfall, the campers across the lake began discharging their weapons. Convinced that the campers were expressing disapproval of their interracial relationship, Dennis returned fire and shot across the lake at the group of patriotic revelors. Fortunately, there were no injuries. Still, Irene continued to convince herself that Dennis was a social drinker who used guns and violence only to protect her from harm.

The First Violent Incident Against Irene

It was February of 2002 when Dennis and his son returned from Alaska. Although Dennis' mother was less than enthusiastic about her son's romantic involvement with a Black woman, she felt obligated to tell Irene the truth. Dennis was not a pilot. Instead, he was unemployed and lived at home with his mother, who also paid for all of his expenses including the costly flying lessons. Dennis also was not a social drinker. He was an alcoholic who had been charged with driving while under the influence, and had been unable to successfully complete any treatment program. Dennis certainly was not a single father. His soon-to-be ex-wife in Texas, whom he had battered in the past, planned to charge him with parental kidnapping for taking their son to Alaska. Finally, Dennis also was not raising his son alone. June, the nanny, provided the majority of child care, also paid for by his mother.

On Valentine's Day, Irene confronted Dennis. "You lied!" she said. He did not deny the truth. "I can't do this!" Irene said, and attempted to leave. Dennis could not accept this response, grabbed Irene, and pleaded with her to stay. When this did not work, he slapped her. In the past, he had yelled and pounded on the furniture, but he had never put his hands on her violently. How could she make sense of this behavior? Irene said, "I took that as he loved me" and "I saw that as 'Please don't leave, I need you.'"

Despite the deception and his violence, Irene tried to salvage the relationship. "You just hope there is going to be a rainbow at the end, and you're going to be the one to find it," she said. Dennis entered yet another alcohol treatment program, but he soon dropped out because he could not believe he had a serious alcohol problem. As a woman of faith, Irene took Dennis to church, which did nothing to change his conduct. For moral support, she even accompanied him to his attorney's office to discuss his pending divorce. Eventually, Irene ran out of hope and options. She stopped taking his calls and tried to occupy herself with the salon and her clients.

Irene's Arrest and Time in Jail

In late March of 2002, Howard called and said, "I need you and Daddy needs you! We miss you real bad." Irene ignored her own internal voice and the advice of three friends that warned her of the impending danger. She decided instead to respond to the child's pleas for attention. It was evident that Dennis still knew how to manipulate Irene. "When he couldn't pull on my heart strings, his son became the heart string puller," she later recalled, although she told herself this would be the last time. Tonight, she would finally end the relationship.

When she arrived, June was on the front porch. As usual, the nanny was drunk. Irene searched for Dennis in the sprawling, suburban home. Howard came out first, jumped into her arms, and then Dennis appeared. Dennis became increasingly belligerent as he watched the interaction between Irene and his son.

After sending the child to his room, Irene tried to leave. Dennis grabbed her by the throat, threw her against the wall, and began choking her. He pulled a gun, put it to her head, and said, "You won't leave me and my son." June, who Dennis had attacked in the past, simply walked away when she observed Dennis' extremely lethal behavior. Irene was then alone, cornered by a large, drunk, angry man who had a weapon. She fought back desperately, was able to break free, and jumped into her car. Dennis followed and began pounding on the hood. As Irene drove away, she watched Dennis dial his cell phone. He yelled after her, "You're going to jail tonight!"

Irene was crying and shaking when she arrived at home. Her neck was hurt and swollen from the strangulation. Initially, she was reluctant to report the assault. "I was just going to take a bath and play like it didn't happen," she said, especially since her experience with two abusive ex-husbands had taught her that batterers could be unpredictable and reporting often made things worse. But Irene also thought, "This man could come over here and finish me off. It's better to be safe, so I called the police." Using a calm and reassuring voice, the 911 operator explained that the police would arrive shortly and take a complete statement.

It was nearly midnight when the police arrived. Dressed in her nightgown and half asleep on the sofa, Irene awoke to heavy footsteps, which "sounded like elephants." "Good, the police are here," she recalled. When she peeked outside the window, the parking lot was "lit up like it was bright morning." She quickly opened the door and six police officers pushed their way into her small apartment. At the time, Irene did not understand why they needed so much manpower to take her statement. After a brief search, four of the officers left. Then Irene was allowed to tell her story:

> God, I'm glad you guys are here. I was at my boyfriend's house and he's got issues and he's been lying to me about being married. He's a drunkard and has a nice son with him. He has all these guns and he tried to choke me and use a gun on me tonight.

The officers seemed to be sympathetic, until one said, "We're sorry, but we have to take you in." While an officer recounted the Miranda rights, she stood up, turned around, and heard the sound of handcuffs closing on her wrists. The charges against her were serious: home invasion, assault and battery with intent to do harm, and possession of an unlicensed firearm.

As he had threatened, Dennis immediately called the police and, according to Irene, told the following story: "My violent, Black girlfriend broke into my house, assaulted me in front of my young son, stole a gun, and took off. See, I even have bruises and June as a witness." As a result, officers from five municipalities were involved in the search for Irene. She then understood the show of force and the search of her apartment. Her heart sank as she argued for her release: "Y'all got it all wrong, he attacked me!" She concluded, "I'm being arrested because I'm a Black woman!" The police denied racial discrimination, and told her that color had nothing to do with it. Dennis had phoned in first, she had been on his property, there was a witness, and there was evidence of an assault. She had to be taken into custody, and the judge could sort things out later.

Irene screamed, cried, and dropped to her knees as the officers escorted her to a waiting patrol car. "I felt like a limp noodle," she said later. She wore a nightgown, with no bra, no panties, no socks, and no shoes. Irene was so afraid that she urinated on herself, which made her legs feel wet and cold. Concerned neighbors peered out of their windows, and watched while the police officers bickered back and forth. Although the assault happened in the suburbs, she lived in the city. Where should she be taken? Finally, they decided to take her to the city jail. She was going to jail–just as Dennis had predicted.

Irene had never been arrested before. She resented being treated like a career criminal. She protested her treatment and immediately began asking questions: "Where do I stand?" "How do you take finger prints?" As a result, she was quickly labeled uncooperative and transferred to solitary confinement. Irene surveyed her dark, dirty surroundings. The thin mattress was filthy, there was blood on the floor, and she listened as the prisoner across the hall banged his head against the cell door.

Yet there was time to reflect on her previous intimate relationships. Her parents had a traditional marriage. Her father worked as a butcher, which enabled him to support the family, and her mother cooked, cleaned, doted on her husband, and raised Irene and her five siblings. However, she was unable to recreate this happy family arrangement. After becoming sexually active, her father, who was a stern disciplinarian, insisted that she get married. So, at age 17 she became the wife of an abusive Black military officer. Irene sought refuge in a battered women's shelter after her first husband threatened her with an ax. In her thirties, she met her second husband at a church function. Although he was a successful Black business man, his physical abuse, heavy drinking, and infidelity eventually ended the marriage.

Interspersed between her two marriages, Irene was involved with several live-in-boyfriends. While there were happy times, there were also arguments, name calling, insults, and physical violence. In most cases, she was the victim. Other times, she verbally abused her partners, and recalled instances where she used violence in retaliation. For example, Irene vandalized one boyfriend's house and car after he had raped her. She shoved another boyfriend down the stairs after he cheated on her. Half jokingly, her mother once called her a "bum magnet." After all, her two Black ex-husbands had been abusive and she had a long history of chaotic relationships. But this was different.

> I was the "bounce back kid" when it came to broken hearts. For once, this was really going to take everything I worked for. It could have took my business. My reputation was on the line. I was embarrassed. I had humiliated my family.

Then, the guard returned and barked, "Are you ready to go through the process?"

She was humble and cooperative. After being strip-searched, she was issued jail underwear, toiletries, and an orange jumpsuit, and then the procedure was over. She was now officially Inmate Number 27. After languishing in jail for two days, it was time for her arraignment. Irene was shackled and moved from the jail to the courthouse. There were two men chained in front and to the back of her. Although it was a short walk, she felt humiliated and prayed that she would not be recognized by a customer, church member, or friend.

After reviewing her case, the judge acknowledged that she had been inappropriately placed with the felons. While the court officials completed the paperwork for her release, Irene was moved to a jail annex that housed inmates who were accused of misdemeanor crimes. This area did not seem as dark and cold, and the guards were friendlier. She said the annex felt like "a cakewalk compared to the other side."

Then, she was released. She carefully gathered and returned all the personal items labeled number 27. In exchange, the guards retrieved her personal property, which included a check for the spare change they had found in her nightgown pocket the night of her arrest. It was late Monday night when she was taken into custody, and she was released at 3:00 o'clock Friday morning. Dressed only in her nightgown, she stood outside of the jailhouse and waited for a friend to pick her up. Although Irene was deeply embarrassed, she was happy to be free.

The Trial

Irene wanted to keep everyone safe, including her customers and other shop owners in the area. However, after multiple visits to the courts, the judge was unwilling to issue a no-contact court order against Dennis. The judge reasoned that Irene was the defendant and supposedly a threat to Dennis. Although Dennis had contacted the courts and asked that the charges be dropped, the prosecutor believed that there was sufficient evidence of an assault and decided to proceed with the case.

"Not guilty!" she asserted at two pre-trial hearings. The court-appointed attorney had an impossible caseload that he could lighten if Irene pled guilty like the other defendants. Irene could not plead guilty, there was just too much to lose. However, she did not have the money to retain a personal lawyer or private investigator, so Irene became an amateur detective. In preparation for the trial, she spent more than $1,000 gathering information such as court transcripts and hospital records. She wanted to prove that Dennis had a long history of alcoholism and violent assaults.

Finally, it was the day of the trial. Her overworked court-appointed attorney had assigned the case to an inexperienced young woman who had recently passed the bar exam. Irene, her friends, and her new lawyer gathered in the hall to devise a plan. I recalled some prior research that suggested that people generally believe that IPV is wrong, yet may feel that it is justified under some circumstances, such as infidelity. Throughout the trial, Irene and the lawyer planned to remind the jury members, who were primarily female, that Dennis had a history of infidelity, alcoholism, and violent assaults against women. We speculated that the jurors would have little sympathy for Dennis and would find Irene not guilty.

The huddle was over and the trial proceeded. As expected, June and Dennis were not credible witnesses. The nanny testified that Irene had broken into the house, jumped on Dennis, and pounded him in the face. Upon cross examination, June reluctantly admitted that she too had once called the police after Dennis had slapped her and spit in her face. Next, Dennis took the witness stand. He looked disheveled and intoxicated. Without making eye contact with the jury members, he repeated the nanny's story in a barely audible voice. Irene's lawyer raised questions about his marital status and alcohol abuse. The prosecuting attorney objected and explained that this information was irrelevant because Dennis was the victim.

Although Irene's freedom was in jeopardy, she was still uncomfortable with this line of questioning. She still cared for Dennis and did not want to see him humiliated in court, even though his violence had resulted in her arrest. During the lunch break, Dennis and June retreated to the parking lot, where the lawyers and jury members observed the pair drinking in Dennis's truck. The damage to their credibility was done. After lunch, the prosecutor called for a mistrial because he claimed the jury could not be fair to his client. The judge was not convinced and ordered that the trial proceed.

Finally, Irene took the stand and told her story. In contrast to Dennis, she was neatly dressed in a business suit, spoke in a humble voice, and made eye contact with jury members. Yes, she had been in his house that night, but she was not a violent intruder. She described the house as a virtual fortress that was well-protected by security gates. She also asked, "How did I beat him down?" After all, he was a large man with easy access to weapons. To conclude her testimony, Irene emphasized that she was actually a victim who had used self-defense. "What they considered me assaulting him was really my trying to get away," she said. She never intended for anyone to be hurt.

Ultimately, there was no need for hospital records, character witnesses, or police reports. The jury quickly returned with a not guilty verdict. After lunch, Dennis and June never returned, so they missed the verdict. However, there was one last court appearance. With the help of another friend, Irene asked a judge for a no-contact order against Dennis. It was granted and Dennis was ordered to avoid future contact with Irene, and he has since complied.

CASE ANALYSIS

The Meeting, Relationship, and IPV

As previously noted, Irene had a long history of violent, chaotic relationships with Black men. Her strong adherence to traditional gender roles may have created the foundation for these abusive relationships. Life histories conducted with Black battered women incarcerated for crimes related to IPV revealed a similar pattern of gender role entrapment (Richie, 1996). More specifically, Irene described herself as a "Daddy's girl" who idolized and romanticized her parent's traditional marriage. Despite her efforts to recreate this family arrangement, she had married and divorced two abusive Black men. Although she was eventually able to extricate herself from these relationships, she continued to believe that women were primarily responsible for maintaining intimate partnerships. Irene hoped that her next relationship, this time involving a White partner, would be different. Gender role entrapment may help to explain why she put the needs of Dennis and his son before her own, and how she could ignore or otherwise explain away the warning signs of escalating violence.

Their rapid and intense relationship was characterized by early expressions of love; however, her friends and relatives were well aware that Dennis had the potential to be extremely dangerous. Although she was reluctant to admit that her life was in danger, there were many indications that Dennis was a potential batterer. For example, he was unemployed, frequently demanded attention, drank heavily, used intimidation and coercive control, and had a fascination with weapons. His level of physical violence, which had increased in severity and frequency from slapping to choking and threats with a weapon, had escalated when Irene attempted to terminate the relationship. These are all risk factors for femicide, which is "the leading cause of death in the United States among young African American women aged 15 to 45 and the seventh leading cause of premature death among women overall" (Campbell et al., 2003, p. 1089).

Irene used self-defense to protect herself from a potentially lethal attack by Dennis, which is consistent with the behavior of other victim-defendants (Melton & Belknap, 2003; Miller, 2001). Although research is limited, it appears that when compared to their White counterparts, Black battered women may have a greater propensity to fight back. This ethnic difference in response to abuse may stem from the frequency and severity of the violence in the lives of Black women, coupled with their historical need to physically defend themselves in order to survive in a society with few systems to protect them. For some Black women, Irene included, their ability to protect themselves was a source of pride and linked to their definition of Black womanhood (Moss, Pitula, Campbell, & Halstead, 1997). As a result, they may not perceive themselves as battered women, even when they sustain serious injury. For example, Johnetta, a 36-year-old woman who had been battered by her husband for nine years, explained:

> Part of the problem is that I am a strong Black woman...so even though he beat me almost to death, I beat him too...by that I'm no regular battered woman, because he got his share of licks. (Richie, 1996, p. 95)

However, the social construction of the "strong Black woman" who fights back is incongruent with the preferred traditional profile of the battered woman as passive, frightened, and helplessly trapped in an abusive relationship. As a result, Black women who use active resistance may receive limited understanding, support, or assistance from others, including the criminal justice system (Richie, 1996).

On the other hand, women's use of violence is not always motivated by self-defense. Sometimes, violence is used in retaliation, as an expression of anger, or as an attempt to gain attention from unresponsive or emotionally unavailable partners. For example, Black women who had been mandated into treatment for IPV offenses were found to be concerned about their partners' infidelity (Henning, Jones, & Holdford, 2005). In addition, they frequently exhibited excessive levels of interpersonal dependency, which is an indicator of an insecure adult attachment style significantly associated with psychological aggression, physical assault, and severe injury to their intimate partners (Carney &

Buttell, 2005). Similar to the research noted above, Irene was often very emotionally dependent on her partners, and the possibility of rejection or infidelity was almost unbearable to her. Consequently, she shoved one boyfriend down the stairs after she discovered his affair, breaking his leg. When his leg healed, he tracked Irene and severely beat her. According to one of Irene's co-workers, his boot prints were visible on her body for days.

Irene may be more appropriately categorized as an example of the "Abused Aggressor" reported by Swan and Snow (2003). In a predominately Black sample, many female IPV perpetrators had initiated violence or injured their partner. Retribution, or getting even with their partners for some actual or perceived misdeed, was a common motive. Despite their violent behavior, these women seldom felt a sense of control, independence, or power within their relationships. Emotionally, they fared almost as poorly as women who had sustained unidirectional male-to-female IPV. In addition, Abused Aggressors tended to suppress their anger and use avoidance as a coping strategy, and reported symptoms of depression, anxiety, and posttraumatic stress. Swan and Snow concluded that "Abused Aggressors may respond to their partners' violence by fighting back with even more violence, but their poor indices of well-being indicate that this strategy does not serve them well" (p. 103).

Arrest, Jail, and Trial

Dennis called the police first, and this gave him the opportunity to proactively define the situation. He described Irene to the police as an armed aggressor who had assaulted him, threatened his family, and fled the scene. Other male IPV perpetrators have also used the "phone first" strategy to manipulate the criminal justice system. In fact, according to one shelter worker in Delaware, "We've had guys wound themselves, cut themselves, and say 'she did it!' and know that she is going to get in trouble and often these are guys who have been perpetrators for some time" (Miller, 2001, p. 1356). This can set the stage for a retaliatory arrest against a victim-defendant after an exaggerated or false complaint is filed by the abuser (Crager et al., 2003).

Despite her ambivalence, however, Irene eventually called the police. While she felt a sense of relief when they arrived, she felt confused, angry, and betrayed when she became one of the growing number of victims arrested for IPV. In fact, a comparison of the number of IPV- related jail bookings for adult female intimates demonstrates an increase from 588 in 1990 to 1,065 in 2000 in the Washington state county where Irene was arrested (Crager et al., 2003).

Irene denied having committed the assault and speculated that the officers' racial bias had resulted in her arrest. There may be some truth to this belief, especially since it is known that compared to their White counterparts, Black women are incarcerated at higher rates for IPV (Simpson et al., 2006). However, Irene's case was nevertheless unique. There was probable cause for an arrest at the scene based on the report from Dennis and a witness (June), as well as the presence of bruises on Dennis's body. In addition, Washington state police officers are required to make an arrest if there is evidence of a domestic assault within the preceding four hours. After the 4-hour mandatory arrest period, an officer has the option to make an arrest or issue a citation (Metropolitan King County Council, 2002). Without proper training, many police officers operating under mandatory arrest procedures may fail to conduct a thorough investigation or miss the obvious signs of a false accusation, and in Irene's case, therefore make an erroneous arrest.

Although Irene's description of her experiences may seem overly dramatic, it is not uncommon. Similar to other victim-defendants (Rajah, Frye, & Haviland, 2006), Irene described being publicly arrested, incarcerated, and shackled as traumatic, painful, and horrifying. At times, she felt transformed from a strong, independent woman to a stigmatized criminal. When she attempted to challenge her maltreatment at the jail, Irene was quickly labeled recalcitrant and placed in solitary confinement. Similar to other marginalized groups, including the mentally ill, people living with HIV, and gang members, this form of institutionally sanctioned isolation has been described as traumatizing and dehumanizing (Shaylor, 1998).

Still, Irene was more fortunate than many others. She had access to financial resources and a strong support system of friends and colleagues. Rather than plead guilty, Irene learned about her rights, gathered information, and went to trial despite her fear and embarrassment. In addition, Irene has since shared her experiences with friends, family members, and business clients in an effort to help other women avoid IPV and possible arrest. Similar to other Black battered women who have participated in research projects (Taylor, 2002), Irene described her testimonial and research involvement as an act of resistance and healing.

Many other battered women may be mystified and intimidated by the criminal justice system, as well as lack the resources available to Irene. If a victim is convicted of an IPV-related crime, she may be forced into a

batterers' treatment program and denied access to victim assistance programs, such as entrance in battered women's shelters or issuance of re-
straining orders. Victims may also incur devastating financial
hardships, such as loss of eligibility for welfare benefits, loss of a job or
housing, and restrictions on employment opportunities in childcare,
teaching, and healthcare. In addition, wrongful convictions may render
many victims ineligible for crime victim compensation and contribute
to loss of child custody to the abuser or the state. Besides the negative
consequences noted above, subsequent threats made by the woman's
abusive partner to report her for probation violations or have her re-ar-
rested also make these victims increasingly vulnerable to future
manipulation and abuse (Crager et al., 2003).

STRATEGIES FOR ADVOCACY

Assisting Black victim-defendants will require collaboration among
researchers, advocates, therapists, and legal professionals such as police
officers, prosecutors, and defense attorneys (for specific suggestions for
each professional group, see Crager et al., 2003; McMahon & Pence,
2003; Osthoff, 2002). Based on the literature, the following
recommendations are offered.

Conduct More Socially-Responsible Research

Although the literature is growing, there needs to be more research
conducted on women who aggress against their intimate partners. More
specifically, scholars in conjunction with victim-defendants and other
stakeholders must develop a more complex model that:

> . . . provides us with a valid and complex understanding of violence
> by women as it takes into account the interactions of antecedents
> (e.g., historical context, social prescriptions of gender roles, social
> and legal reactions) as well as immediate conditions and conse-
> quences (e.g., early socialization, individual experiences, inten-
> tions, partner's responses, repercussions on the individual as well as
> work and family) of such actions. (Dasgupta, 2002, p. 1376)

For Black women, such theoretical models should explore their use
of violence within the intersections of race, gender, and social class
(Swan & Snow, 2006).

Identify the Primary Aggressor

Service providers should work harder to identify the primary aggressor. This would require asking difficult questions such as: Who uses violence? When? What kinds of violence do they use-physical, sexual, psychological, coercive control? What are the motivations, intent, and outcome of the violence? (Osthoff, 2002).

Professionals should also consider the history of abuse, prior medical records, past police reports, the presence of protective orders, 911 tapes, neighbor and witness statements, and injuries. For example, if a victim is being strangled or restrained, she may bite or scratch her batterer to get away. In contrast, victim bruises due to strangulation may not be visible immediately, especially on dark-skinned women. Consequently, when the police arrive, the batterer may present with very visible scratches or bite marks while the victim does not, possibly resulting in victim arrest if officers are not aware of such common injury patterns (Crager et al., 2003). With Black women, it would also be quite important to challenge the myth that they are inherently more violent than women from other ethnic groups. Some Black women are socialized to fight back, and sometimes they may injure their partners; however, they may not be the primary aggressors (Moss et al., 1997).

Offer Appropriate Services

Women who are arrested (Henning et al., 2006) or in treatment (Miller & Meloy, 2006; Swan & Snow, 2002) for IPV are not homogenous groups. While a small number of women are indeed the primary aggressor within their relationships, other women engage in mutual aggression, and some have never been violent within an intimate relationship prior to the incident that led to their arrest. Assuming that women arrested for IPV form a heterogeneous group, services should be tailored to individual needs. For example, victim-defendants and/or women who are engaged in bidirectional asymmetrical violence should receive safety planning and access to support services such as emergency shelters, affordable housing, and transportation. Legal advocacy to expunge erroneous convictions should also be considered. In contrast, the small number of women who appear to be primary perpetrators may need programs that challenge their attitudes toward violence and reduce their minimization, denial, and externalization of blame for their offenses (Henning et al.; Miller & Meloy).

Even though there are successful treatment programs for women convicted of IPV offenses (e.g., Larance, 2006; Miller & Meloy, 2006), their numbers are few and the development of such programs is still in its infancy. However, the literature that is available suggests that curricula should be developed with the awareness that many women in batterer treatment programs have had previous victim-related exposure to violence, and may experience anxiety, depression, and post-traumatic stress disorder. Many other women face serious life challenges, including unemployment, lack of transportation and housing, child care problems, and ongoing substance use (Miller & Meloy). Furthermore, Black battered women are somewhat more likely to be enrolled in programs for batterers, even though they have high rates of past trauma and have accessed victim services in the past (Abel, 2001). Consequently, therapists and advocates should consider how class and race discrimination can create additional challenges for Black women (Loy, Machen, Beaulieu, & Greif, 2005; McAdory, 2005).

To conclude, I am aware that proponents on both sides of the gender symmetry debate can find evidence to support their position. For instance, those who believe that women are equally as violent as men and should be treated accordingly by the criminal legal system will see Irene's experience as evidence that mandatory/proarrest laws are being applied properly. Those arguing that IPV is a gender-based crime with primarily female victims and male offenders may highlight the severity of the violence directed toward Irene. There is also the danger of reinforcing stereotypes about the inherent violent nature of Black women by focusing on Irene. Ultimately, anti-violence activists, mental health service providers, shelter workers, and researchers must engage in candid discussions about the complexity of women's use of IPV and therefore move past a polarized debate, especially for Black women. Hopefully, if we can begin to grapple with this difficult topic, fewer victim-defendants will hear the words: "Sorry, we have to take you in."

REFERENCES

Abel, E. M. (2001). Comparing the social services utilization, exposure to violence, and trauma symptomology of domestic violence female "victims" and female "batterers." *Journal of Family Violence, 16*, 401-420.

Archer, J. (2000). Sex differences in aggression between heterosexual partners: A meta-analytic review. *Psychological Bulletin, 126*, 651-680.

Benson, M. L., & Fox, G. L. (2004). *When violence hits home: How economics and neighborhood play a role* (NCJ 205004). Washington, DC: National Institute of Justice. Retrieved November 12, 2006 from http://www.ncjrs.gov/pdffiles1/nij/205004.pdf

Bible, A., Dasgupta, S., & Osthoff, S. (Eds.). (2002-2003). Women's use of violence in intimate relationships: Part 1, 2, 3 [Special issues]. *Violence Against Women, 8*(11/12) & *9*(1).

Buttell, F. P., & Carney, M. M. (Eds.) (2006). *Women who perpetrate relationship violence: Moving beyond political correctness.* Binghamton, NY: Haworth Press.

Caetano, R., Ramisetty-Mikler, S., & Field, C. A. (2005). Unidirectional and bidirectional intimate partner violence among White, Black, and Hispanic couples in the United States. *Violence and Victims, 20,* 393-404.

Campbell, J. C., Webster, D., Koziol-McLain, J., Block, C., Campbell, D., Curry, M. A. et al. (2003). Risk factors for femicide in abusive relationships: Results from a multisite case control study. *American Journal of Public Health, 93,* 1089-1097.

Carney, M. M. & Buttell, F. P. (2005). Exploring the relevance of attachment theory as a dependent variable in the treatment of women mandated into treatment for domestic violence offenses. In F. P. Buttell, & M. M. Carney (Eds.), *Women who perpetrate relationship violence: Moving beyond political correctness* (pp. 33-61). Binghamton, NY: Haworth Press.

Clark, M. L., Beckett, J., Wells, M., & Dungee-Anderson, D. (1994). Courtship violence among African American college students. *Journal of Black Psychology, 20,* 264-281.

Crager, M., Cousin, M., & Hardy, T. (2003). *Victim-Defendants: An emerging challenge in responding to domestic violence in Seattle and the King County Region.* Seattle, WA: King County Coalition Against Domestic Violence. Retrieved August 15, 2006 from http://www.mincava.umn.edu/documents/victimdefendant/victimdefendant.pdf

Cunradi, C. B., Caetano, R., Clark, C., & Schafer, J. (1999). Alcohol-related problems and intimate partner violence among White, Black, and Hispanic couples in the U.S. *Alcoholism: Clinical and Experimental Research, 23,* 1492-1501.

Cunradi, C. B., Caetano, R., Clark, C., & Schafer, J. (2000). Neighborhood poverty as a predictor of intimate partner violence among White, Black, and Hispanic couples in the United States: A multilevel analysis. *Annals of Epidemiology, 10,* 297-308.

Cunradi, C. B., Caetano, R., & Schafer, J. (2002). Socioeconomic predictors of intimate partner violence among White, Black, and Hispanic couples in the United States. *Journal of Family Violence, 17,* 377-389.

Dasgupta, D. S. (2002). A framework for understanding women's use of nonlethal violence in intimate heterosexual relationships. *Violence Against Women, 8,* 1364-1389.

DeLeon-Granados, W., Wells, W., & Binsbacher, R. (2006). Arresting developments: Trends in female arrests for domestic violence and proposed explanations. *Violence Against Women, 12,* 355-371.

Dugan, L., Nagin, D., & Rosenfeld, R. (2003). Exposure reduction or retaliation? The effects of domestic violence resources on intimate partner homicide. *Law & Society, 27,* 169-198.

Dutton, D. G., Nicholls, T. L., & Spidel, A. (2005). Female perpetrators of intimate abuse. In F. P. Buttell, & M. M. Carney (Eds.), *Women who perpetrate relationship violence: Moving beyond political correctness* (pp. 1-31). Binghamton, NY: Haworth Press.

Feder, L., & Henning, K. (2005). A comparison of male and female dually arrested domestic violence offenders. *Violence and Victims, 20,* 153-171.

Field, C. A., & Caetano, R. (2005). Longitudinal model predicting mutual partner violence among White, Black, and Hispanic couples in the United States general population. *Violence and Victims, 20,* 499-511.

Fox, J. A., & Zawitz, M. W. (2006). *Homicide trends in the United States.* Washington, DC: U.S. Department of Justice, Bureau of Justice Statistics. Retrieved January 3, 2007 from, http://www.ojp.usdoj.gov/bjs/homicide/intimates.htm

Hamberger, L. K. (2005). Men's and women's use of intimate partner violence in clinical samples: Toward a gender-sensitive analysis. *Violence and Victims, 20,* 131-151.

Hampton, R. L., Gelles, R. J., & Harrop, J. W. (1989). Is violence in Black families increasing? A comparison of 1975 and 1985 national survey rates. *Journal of Marriage and the Family, 51,* 969-980.

Henning, K., & Feder, L. (2004). A comparison of men and women arrested for domestic violence: Who presents the greater threat? *Journal of Family Violence, 19,* 69-80.

Henning, K., Jones, A. R., & Holdford, R. (2005). "I didn't do it, but if I did I had a good reason": Minimization, denial, and attributions of blame among male and female domestic violence offenders. *Journal of Family Violence, 20,* 131-139.

Henning, K., Renauer, B., & Holdford, R. (2006). Victim or offender? Heterogeneity among women arrested for intimate partner violence. *Journal of Family Violence, 21,* 351-368.

Kimmel, M. S. (2002). "Gender symmetry" in domestic violence: A substantive and methodological research review. *Violence Against Women, 8,* 1332-1363.

Larance, L. Y. (2006). Serving women who use force in their intimate heterosexual relationships: An extended view. *Violence Against Women, 12,* 622-640.

Lockhart, L., & White, B. W. (1989). Understanding marital violence in the Black community. *Journal of Interpersonal Violence, 4,* 421-436.

Loy, E., Machen, L., Beaulieu, M., & Greif, G. L. (2005). Common themes in clinical work with women who are domestically violent. *The American Journal of Family Therapy, 33,* 33-44.

McAdory, D. D. (2005). Black women victims and perpetrators of domestic violence: A therapeutic model incorporating racism and Black history. In M. Rastogi & E. Wieling (Eds.), *Voices of color: First-person account of ethnic minority therapists* (pp. 255-264). Thousand Oaks, CA: Sage Publications.

McMahon, M., & Pence, E. (2003). Making social change: Reflections on individual and institutional advocacy with women arrested for domestic violence. *Violence Against Women, 9,* 47-74.

Melton, H. C., & Belknap, J. (2003). He hits, she hits: Assessing gender differences and similarities in officially reported intimate partner violence. *Criminal Justice and Behavior, 30,* 328-348.

Metropolitan King County Council. (2002). *Domestic and dating violence: An information and resource handbook.* Retrieved December 3, 2006 from, http://www.metrokc.gov/mkcc/docs/dvint.pdf

Miller, N. (2004). *Domestic violence: A review of state legislation defining police and prosecution duties and powers.* Alexandria, VA: Institute for Law and Justice.

Miller, S. L. (2001). The paradox of women arrested for domestic violence: Criminal justice professionals and service providers respond. *Violence Against Women, 7,* 1339-1376.

Miller, S. L. (2003). Arrest policies for domestic violence: Their implications for battered women. In R. Muraskin (Ed.), *It's a crime: Women and justice* (pp. 307-329). Upper Saddle River, NJ: Prentice Hall.

Miller, S. L. (2005). *Victims as offenders: The paradox of women's violence in relationships.* New Brunswick, NJ: Rutgers University Press.

Miller, S. L., & Meloy, M. L. (2006). Women's use of force: Voices of women arrested for domestic violence. *Violence Against Women, 12,* 89-115.

Moss, V. A., Pitula, C. R., Campbell, J. C., & Halstead, L. (1997). The experience of terminating an abusive relationship from an Anglo and African American perspective: A qualitative descriptive study. *Issues in Mental Health Nursing, 18,* 433-454.

Osthoff, S. (2002). But, Gertrude, I beg to differ, a hit is not a hit is not a hit: When battered women are arrested for assaulting their partners. *Violence Against Women, 8,* 1521-1544.

Potter, H. (2006). An argument for Black feminist criminology: Understanding African American women's experiences with intimate partner abuse using an integrated approach. *Feminist Criminology, 1,* 106-124.

Rajah, V., Frye, V., & Haviland, M. (2006). "Aren't I a victim?": Notes on identity challenges relating to police action in a mandatory arrest jurisdiction. *Violence Against Women, 12,* 897-916.

Rajan, M., & McCloskey, K. (2007). Victims of intimate partner violence: Arrest rates across recent studies. *Journal of Aggression, Maltreatment, & Trauma, 15*(3/4), 27-52.

Richie, B. E. (1996). *Compelled to crime: The gender entrapment of battered Black women.* New York: Routledge.

Rosen, L. N. (2006). Origin and goals of the "Gender Symmetry" workshop. *Violence Against Women, 12,* 997-1002.

Shaylor, C. (1998). "It's like living in a black hole": Women of color and solitary confinement in the prison industrial complex. *New England Journal on Criminal and Civil Confinement, 24,* 385-416.

Simpson, S. S., Bouffard, L. A., Garner, J., & Hickman, L. (2006). The influence of legal reform on the probability of arrest in domestic violence cases. *Justice Quarterly, 23,* 297-316.

Swan, S. C., & Snow, D. L. (2002). A typology of women's use of violence in intimate relationships. *Violence Against Women, 8,* 286-319.

Swan, S. C., & Snow, D. L. (2003). Behavioral and psychological differences among abused women who use violence in intimate relationships. *Violence Against Women, 9,* 75-109.

Swan, S. C., & Snow, D. L. (2006). The development of a theory of women's use of violence in intimate relationships. *Violence Against Women, 12*, 1026-1045.

Taylor, J. Y. (2002). Talking back: Research as an act of resistance and healing for African American women survivors of intimate male partner violence. In C. M. West (Ed.), *Violence in the lives of Black women: Battered, black, and blue* (pp. 145-160). Binghamton, NY: The Haworth Press.

Temple, J. R., Weston, R., & Marshall, L. L. (2005). Physical and mental health outcomes of women in nonviolent, unilaterally violent, and mutually violent relationships. *Violence and Victims, 20*, 335-359.

Websdale, N. (2001). *Policing the poor: From slave plantation to public housing.* Boston: Northeastern University Press.

West, C. M. & Rose, S. (2000). Dating aggression among low-income African American youth. *Violence Against Women, 6*, 470-494.

Submitted: December 9, 2004
Revised: January 19, 2007
Revised: May 4, 2007
Accepted: May 26, 2007

CULTURAL AND ENVIRONMENTAL INFLUENCES

Non-Violent Survival Strategies in the Face of Intimate Partner Violence and Economic Discrimination

Dana-Ain Davis

Intimate partner violence (IPV) is defined by the National Center for Injury Prevention and Control (NCIPC) as actual or threatened physical or sexual violence or psychological and emotional abuse directed toward a spouse, ex-spouse, current or former boyfriend or girlfriend, or current or former dating partner. Intimate partners may be heterosexual or of the same sex (Salzman, Fanslow, McMahon, & Shelley, 1999). The NCIPC's definition is problematic because in defining IPV it draws on a family systems model, suggesting that men and women perpetrate violence and are victimized at equal rates. Alternatively and more appropriately, a feminist analysis of IPV takes into account gendered norms, power differentials, and external forces that contextualize victimization (e.g., poverty). In other words, the latter perspective argues that women are the primary victims of the violence and challenges the seemingly gender-neutral experience of IPV. The case that IPV exists at equal rates among men and women relies on a number of studies, usually survey data, which have shown that women perpetrate violence as often as men do. For example, the National Family Violence Survey (Straus & Gelles, 1986) of 3,520 men and women found that one year prior to the survey, 12.5% of wives self-reported that they used violence against their husbands compared to 11.3% of husbands. O'Leary et al. (1989) found that among newlyweds, women reported they were more likely to use severe violence than were men. Another study by Strauss (1999) shows that women self report physical aggression as often as

Archer (1999) reviews the evidence supporting equal rates of ~~en~~ and women. Critiques of these studies suggest that they often fail to explore the antecedents, motivations, contexts, or consequences of the violence, often resulting in the presumption of the "mutuality of violence" (Johnson & Ferraro, 2000).

Adding fuel to the debate regarding women's role as primary IPV perpetrators are data regarding IPV arrests. Women are being arrested in increasing numbers as a consequence of mandatory arrest legislation enacted in several states in the 1980s and 1990s.[1] The view that women are equally responsible in the IPV dynamic has been buttressed by data showing increased arrests of women. For example, Goldberg (1999) reported a surge in arrests of women in many states across the country. As evidence, he noted that in Vermont 23% of domestic assault arrests are women and that as a result of mandatory arrest, women's arrests in California rose from 5% in 1987 to 15% in 1997. However, others have argued that the assumption that women engage in acts of aggression as often as men as "proven" by arrest data does not factor in that when women are arrested, police often have not made a distinction between the victim and primary aggressor (Martin, 1997; O'Dell, this issue; Sheffield, 1995; Worden & Pollitz, 1984). Thus, while women may be aggressive, they are not usually the initiator of violence. One attempt to clarify the confusion over IPV-related arrests was underscored by New York Governor George Pataki's comments at the 1997 signing ceremony for New York's Primary Aggressor law formulated in response to women being arrested for fighting back. Governor Pataki noted that women victimized by domestic violence should not be revictimized through the arrest process when they defend themselves (Clifford, 1999). Although women no doubt engage in aggressive behavior, it is clear that the definition of IPV leads to a misinterpretation of women's use of violence. The problem with the traditional definition of IPV is the focus on women's isolated behavioral acts that can divert attention away from the fact that many women are the primary victims of abuse. There is also the need to consider what else battered women do in response to violence besides using violence to protect themselves. Many women employ mechanisms other than retaliation to deal with the violence in their lives. One strategy is the use of welfare to help them escape violent abusers. This is especially the case for poor women, where the context of poverty complicates their efforts to leave battering relationships.

According to the U.S. Census Bureau, there are about 36 million poor people living in the United States. In 2004, a family with three people (one adult and two dependent children) would be considered living in poverty if their household income was $15,219 (National Poverty Center, n.d.). However, that family of three is likely to be composed of a woman and two children because women are 40% more likely to be poor than men, situating poverty as a gender issue (NOW Legal Defense and Education Fund, 2004). Furthermore, violence is pervasive in the lives of poor and low-income women suggesting that there is a connection between poverty and violence. Supporting evidence comes from Rennison and Welchans (2000), who produced a report indicating that women living in households with lower annual incomes experience violence seven times greater than women living in households with the highest annual household income (20 per 1,000 versus 3 per 1,000). These findings point to the need to explore factors impinging upon the lives of battered women. In response to the violence in their lives, many women do not resort to violence, but rather use welfare as one alternative mechanism for leaving violent relationships. In fact, according to Lyon (2002), access to independent economic resources, including welfare, is central to abused women's decision-making and safety planning (also see Brandwein, 1999a; Davies, Lyon, & Monti-Catania, 1998; Raphael, 1995).

This article examines the intersection of poverty and violence, suggesting that women often use welfare as a way to deal with IPV. In the face of IPV and economic hardship, women strategize their survival to remain free of violence and achieve economic security. Case studies that situate poverty and violence as relational phenomena will be presented, and four strategies women utilize to keep intimate and economic oppression in abeyance will be identified. An analysis of the racialized dimension of the use of these strategies is presented, followed by a discussion of how women's responses to IPV and economic discrimination overlap.

In teasing out women's responses to IPV, most studies have assumed, a priori, a particularly neutral gender/power stance, de-emphasizing the exceptionally high rates of poverty and violence against women. As an alternative, this article draws on anthropological methods and seeks to broaden the discussion of IPV by examining alternatives to violence used by women within the context of poverty and welfare. Given that women are situated differentially from men in economic terms, violence and poverty are viewed as correlational, not necessarily causal, and both engender a range of reactions. The present effort views the intersecting issues of violence, poverty, and welfare access as circumstances that generate an assortment of responses by women as a means to alleviate the intimate and structural violence of poverty in their lives.

This study is not unique in its critique of the context of IPV research approaches, particularly its focus on violent women, how measurement choice influences research findings, and motivations and antecedents in women's aggression (Cook, 2002). Several researchers have produced analyses that de-essentialize and de-contextualize IPV in general and women's aggression in particular. Bohannon, Dosser, and Lindley (1995) documented discrepancies in self reported information, while O'Leary, Vivian, and Malone (1992) noted deviations in self-disclosure depending on whether reports are collected in oral vs. written form. Swan and Snow (2002) interviewed 108 low-income women who had used physical violence against a male intimate partner and developed a typology of women's violence in intimate relationships. Their findings reveal that women's abusive relationships vary along dimensions of physical abuse and control, and that women aggressors are less violent overall in relationships than those in which male partners are aggressors. Leisring, Dowd, and Rosenbaum (2003) argued that there are specific characteristics of partner-aggressive women, a finding that has implications for treatment, especially the need for different treatment modalities for female and male aggressive partners. Another review examined differences between male and female IPV, specifically noting distinctions in "genderized" reactions (Malloy, McCloskey, Grigsby, & Gardner, 2003). Nuanced analyses of this type broadly reveal the differential physical, psychological, and emotional impacts of IPV for women vs. men. The most congruent finding across these critiques is that women experience significant violence from their partners, even in relationships in which they are the primary aggressors. The question this article raises is: "What other strategies, other than striking back, might women employ in the face of IPV victimization?"

Although a number of studies lead us toward understanding the complex dynamics involved, the phrase "intimate partner violence" still conveys an assumption that violence is impacted only by factors located within an intimate relationship. This premise limits what one looks for as a response to violence and presumes women respond only to intimate forms of violence, when in fact their responses are also influenced by both poverty and policy, particularly the policy of welfare reform. Welfare reform is the popular phrase used to describe the Personal Responsibility and Work Opportunity Reconciliation Act of 1996 (PRWORA), signed by President Clinton in August 1996. The Act created a new program, Temporary Assistance to Needy Families (TANF), that eliminated the federal guarantee of public assistance and shifted the responsibility of providing assistance from the federal government to the states. The Act made assistance programs time-limited; a person may now only receive assistance for a lifetime of five years, whereas in the past people received assistance when they needed it. The Act also requires recipients to work or be engaged in work-related activities under threat of being sanctioned or losing their benefits if they do not comply with work requirements.

The links between IPV, poverty, and welfare reform policy have been examined by a number of researchers. According to Kurz (1999), poor women who wish to leave violent relationships face many barriers to achieving economic stability. She notes that government assistance is crucial, and the fact that women use welfare to leave violent relationships suggests this too is a response to IPV. However, recent shifts in welfare and other poverty-related policies make it difficult for battered women to achieve safety and economic autonomy. For example, changes in public housing policy, specifically the Housing Opportunity Program Extension Act of 1996, shifted the authority of particular public housing policies from the federal to the local level. Prior to the Extension Act, battered women were given preference for receiving federal housing assistance. Now, however, no such federal policy is in place (U.S. Department of Housing and Urban Development, 1997). A "one strike policy" for eviction now also exists; that is, public housing authorities are allowed to deny housing and evict residents based on a zero tolerance policy. While this policy is directed at decreasing gang and drug activity, some battered women are being evicted if police are called to their house too many times (Renzetti, 2001).

These policies may be viewed as forms of structural violence, a term taken from peace theorist Galtung (1969). According to Galtung, structural violence refers to existing constraints on human potential due to economic and political structures. An anthropological elaboration of that definition has been offered by Anglin (1998), who argued that structural violence exists when institutions expose people to hazards that can impede one's well-being. She further noted that changes in government policies, such as welfare reform, represent one form of structural violence by withdrawing social support from the "undeserving" in an attempt to resolve local and national budgetary problems. Thus, we may view these complex intersecting issues as violence that "expropriates vital economic and non-material resources, subverting chances for survival" (p. 145). Consequently, women respond not only to IPV but to precarious economic circumstances and policies in various

ways. One example of how the denial of vital resources subverts battered women's choices vis a vis survival is expressed in Sherita's case.[2]
Sherita is a 38-year old Black woman who was victimized by her drug
abusing boyfriend, Joey. His violent behavior increased after she lost
her job due to lack of transportation.

> We could be talking like you and I right now, sitting across from
> each other. He'd be getting high, he'd be calm, cool, and collected.
> And then he would snap. I might go into the bathroom and he'd
> follow me, close the door, and next thing I know I'm on the
> floor...I had to get out of that apartment...I moved in with a couple
> upstairs.

Sherita did not fight back, but went to the Department of Social Services to see if she could secure housing and financial assistance to leave
Joey. However, the fact that Sherita had previously lost a job made her
ineligible for assistance and she was sanctioned for 90 days. Within that
90-day period, as she waited for the sanction to be lifted, Joey beat
Sherita, splitting her lip and her eye as well as dislodging several teeth.
She continued to work with Social Services to achieve safety, in spite of
policies that put her at risk for further abuse. Ultimately, she entered
Angel House, a shelter for battered women, although that was not her
first chosen strategy to attempt to end the violence in her life.

This example captures a different response to IPV and sheds light on
how constructing violence as gender neutral obscures two important issues. First, women experience a range of violence within intimate and
structural spheres; in Sherita's case, from both Joey and the lack of federal and local assistance. Second, many women like Sherita engage in
non-violent responses to IPV that often precede, or more likely substitute for, women's use of physical aggression against intimates. According to Sherita, she had not struck back at her abuser.

Economic fragility is clearly an important issue in women's IPV experiences, and I will explore some of the responses battered women had
to violence, poverty, and policy. In so doing, this article critiques the
"gender-neutral discourse" often present in the IPV literature, and instead builds on literature that documents the linkage between violence
and welfare use. The intent of this effort is not to test theories or suggest
causal relationships. Rather, my intent is to show that women employ a
variety of strategies in response to IPV that intersect with their responses to poverty, and to suggest that women engage in many
strategies other than resorting to violence.

METHODS

Participants

This article is based on a nearly two year (February 1998 to December 2000) qualitative study of 22 women living in Angel House, a battered women's shelter located in Laneville (River Valley County, New York), where women are permitted to live no more than 90 days. In interviews that lasted 6-12 hours, women discussed their life histories, experiences with violence, and use of welfare resources.

Whites comprised 41% of the entire shelter resident population, Blacks 33%, Latinas 18%, Asians 2%, and 7% were Other. However, because the goal was to learn more about Black women's experiences with violence, poverty, and welfare reform, the racial/ethnic breakdown of study participants was somewhat different than the overall shelter population. Of the 22 women interviewed, 13 were Black (59%), 4 White (18%), 3 Latina (14%), 1 Asian (5%), and 1 Indian (5%). Moreover, while the average shelter resident had less than 12 years of education, the average study participant had a high school diploma, some college, or vocational training.

Besides the inverted Black/White demographic and differences in academic levels, all other characteristics of the study participants and the general shelter population were comparable. The average shelter resident and study participant was between the ages of 30 and 39, most were single with children, and most had household incomes of less than $9,999 at the time of shelter entry. Table 1 summarizes participant characteristics. The women in the study were also demographically similar to the national welfare caseload. Generally, about 90% of TANF recipients are women. In 2000, national data showed that the average age of a welfare recipient was 31 years old and about half had a formal education of 12 years or more. In terms of race, 31% of the national welfare caseload was White, 39% were Black, and 22% were Hispanic (U.S. Department of Health and Human Services, 2004).

Approach

During this research project, the overall goal was to analyze the impact of welfare reform on the lives of battered Black women living in Laneville, NY. Laneville is a small city in NY State, which limits the applicability of findings to that particular geographic location and to the women who were interviewed. Thus, the impact of welfare reform and

TABLE 1. 1999 Comparative Demographics: Angel House (AH) Clients vs. Study Participants (Study)

	AH *N*	AH %*	Study *N*	Study %
Total Women	125	100%	22	100%
AGE GROUP				
<=19	10	8%	4	18%
20-29	45	36%	4	18%
30-39	48	38%	11	50%
40-49	20	16%	2	9%
50-59	2	2%	1	5%
Unknown	--	--	--	--
ETHNICITY				
White	51	41%	4	18%
Black	41	33%	13	59%
Latina	22	18%	3	14%
Asian	2	2%	1	5%
Other	9	7%	1	5%
INCOME LEVEL				
None	39	31%	2†	9%
Under 9,999	66	53%	13	59%
10-14,999	14	11%	1	5%
15-21,999	3	2%	2	9%
22-29,000	0	0	0	0
30,000+	3	2%	0	14%
Unknown	0	0	1	5%
CITIZENSHIP				
U.S. Citizen	109	87%	13	59%
Documented	11	9%	6	27%
Undocumented	5	4%	1	5%
Unclear	0	0	2	9%
EDUCATION				
<12 years	46	37%	4	18%
H.S./GED	34	27%	8	36%
Some College	23	18%	2	9%
College Grad	17	14%	2	9%
Vocational	3	2%	5	23%
Unknown	2	2%	1	5%
MARITAL STATUS				
Single	66	53%	14	64%
Married	39	31%	5	23%
Separated	9	7%	3	14%
Divorced	8	6%	0	0%
Widowed	3	2%	0	0%

*Percentages may add up to more than 100 due to rounding.
† Both individuals were students and had no reportable income.
Source of Angel House Data: 1999 Shelter Statistics Report.
AH – Angel House total population.
Study – study sample.

battered women's responses to it are not necessarily generalizable to rural areas (see Websdale [1998] for further information concerning rural poverty and IPV). The present research examined four dimensions of social life under welfare reform policy: (a) interactions with Department of Social Service caseworkers, (b) meeting work requirements and training mandates, (c) accessing housing,

(d) and accessing childcare. In analyzing life histories and interviews, active economic-related strategies emerged that appeared to be a consequence of changes in welfare policy that mandates work or work-related activity within the context of having been battered (Davis, 2006). The research design included participant observation, structured interviews, life history interviews, and case record review. Over the course of two years, I observed behavior by participating in the daily activities and life events of women in the sample. Women were accompanied to appointments at Social Services, during trips to find housing and employment, and during social visits in their homes after having left the shelter. Maintaining contact with most study participants allowed me to spend intensive time with women and observe them over time, a hallmark of the ethnographic enterprise (e.g., Websdale, 1998). In contrast to traditional survey approaches that tend to solidify identities and experiences as they appear at one point in time, ethnographic methods represent people's lives as a process that unfolds over time (Susser, 1996).

Life histories were conducted with the battered women following the structured interviews. The life history interview is an excellent ethnographic method that facilitates delving into the intimate spheres of people's lives, and allows researchers to illuminate events that shape people's experiences. To validate demographic data, life history data, and institutional relations, case record reviews were also conducted. Case records are kept at the shelter and contain pertinent information regarding reasons for coming to the shelter, copies of important documents needed to apply for public assistance, and on-going documentation of women's shelter exit strategies and life plans.

In addition, 40 personnel from battered women's and poor people's advocacy centers, personnel at community-based organizations, staff at both the Department of Social Services and Department of Labor, and other state-based agencies were interviewed.

Procedures

Women were recruited from among those living at Angel House. Shelter staff announced the research project at weekly House meetings, and those interested made contact with the researcher. Women also became part of the project upon recommendations from other women who had already been interviewed. Thus, women were self-selected for participation.

RESULTS

Poverty and Violence

A major contextual variable in understanding IPV is the issue of so-cioeconomic status. Although women in all socioeconomic groups ex-perience IPV, financial stress, poverty, and living in poor neighborhoods are associated with higher levels of violent crime, in-cluding IPV (Browne, Salomon, & Bassuk, 1999; Stark & Flitcraft, 1988). In addition, a number of studies since 1995 have documented the prevalence of violence in the lives of low-income women, especially those on welfare (e.g., Brandwein, 1999b; Brown & Bassuk, 1997). Embedded in these studies is the claim that women use welfare as a re-sponse to IPV. In other words, in order to leave violent relationships, some women utilize welfare to escape.

Jocelyn is a 36-year-old White woman who left her husband, Gus, af-ter an "accident" from which she received a broken arm and jaw, head trauma, and unspecified nerve damage. Although she had lived a mate-rially comfortable life–Gus earned in excess of $50,000 as a police offi-cer and they owned their own home–Jocelyn wanted to finish college and Gus refused to pay for it. The "accident" happened shortly after she took a job cleaning houses to pay for her own education. Subsequently, Jocelyn left Gus and reported that she had: "...no source of income and am unable to work. I am not eligible for unemployment since I have been working off the books cleaning houses. I need welfare." While Jocelyn was not poor in terms of overall household income, she lacked an independently earned income that made her economically reliant on her husband. The dissolution of their relationship rendered her poor, and she needed government assistance for the purpose of her own phys-ical and economic survival. Other similar examples are discussed below.

Strategizing Survival in the Face of IPV and Economic Violence

Women want to live lives free of violence, and they often take cre-ative steps to achieve that goal. In their protective trajectory, leaving their batterers is but one step. Fifty percent of all women in the present sample stated they were using public assistance as a strategy to escape violent relationships. They had applied for food stamps and planned to draw on social service assistance in an effort to create separate house-holds. Upon entry into a shelter, women in the state of New York apply for social services. However, as of 1997, these women also are mandated to meet the requirements of the PRWORA in exchange for receiving assistance. Although battered women are afforded some protection against the mandates of welfare reform through waivers provided by the Family Violence Option,[3] there has been uneven application of this waiver (see Hearn, 2000; Raphael, 1999) and many of the women interviewed in this study were unable to use it effectively. Consequently, the multiple barriers imposed by welfare policy, such as benefit loss, food stamp reduction, structural inability to secure employment at a living wage, and lack of affordable housing, could all prompt some women to return to their batterers. In these case studies, however, women who faced structural barriers during or after applying for welfare tried to negotiate obstacles while ensuring their own safety and that of their children. Limited access to resources and fear of having to return to violent men precipitated women's development of alternatives to become both safe and make ends meet. In the absence of realizing financial security through state funds due to sanctioning, case closure, and benefit reductions, women took action to neutralize fluctuations in the availability of economic resources.

How do women who are battered and poor survive the increased poverty and displacement brought about by IPV as well as policy sanctions? I found that during and after the shelter experience, when situated in their own homes, women experienced financial, housing, and child-care vulnerability because government assistance was conditional and was no longer a safety net. Since poor women have rarely been able to survive on institutional income-transfers alone, they have historically had to construct survival strategies. Four strategies, each of which will be defined and elaborated upon below, emerged as patterns in this study and each served to help women recreate stable households and families in light of policies and structural constraints. These were: (a) the use of speech acts where women tried to talk their way into securing economic resources, primarily from governmental institutional personnel such as caseworkers at the Department of Social Services; (b) the creation of fictive kin support networks where women developed familial-like relationships with people in their social networks that they had met while living at the shelter and who were expected to help women out in times of need; (c) initiating instrumental relationships where women provided a "favor" and then drew on the obligation of reciprocity to get what they needed; and (d) engaging in "illegalities," where women did something either outside the law or outside "normative" standards of feminine behavior. While each strategy is discussed independently below, this in no way suggests that women employed only one strategy at a time. Often, they used as many strategies simultaneously as were necessary. Table 2 summarizes strategies women used to address the lack of access to material needs differentiated by race.

Of the 22 study participants, 16 (72%) used at least one of the four strategies identified. Of the six women who did not engage in any of the strategies, two were non-English speakers and may not have used these types of strategic skills due to language and/or cultural barriers. One Asian woman with a lot of economic resources did not require additional assistance, and thus did not use any of the strategies. There are no clear reasons why the remaining three did not employ any strategy at all. However, a common factor among these three was that they were all 19 years of age at the time of their shelter stay, and it is possible that utilizing these strategies requires a certain level of maturity and possession of life-skills.

It should also be noted that of the 22 women interviewed, three women completed only partial interviews due to short shelter stays. The partial interviews did not preclude them from revealing strategies they used; therefore, sufficient data were collected to justify their inclusion in the analysis. Given that women often used more than one strategy, the frequency with which each strategy was deployed and the percent of women in each racial/ethnic group who employed that strategy is noted in Table 2. Thus, an individual woman may be counted more than once if she used more than one strategy.

Race and the Use of Strategies

Although not all of the Black women used all of the strategies, all strategies were used by Black women, more than women of any other racial/ethnic group. Across race, Black and White women were equally likely to use speech acts and fictive kin. Both Black and White women used speech acts the most, followed by fictive kin. Latina women used only fictive kin to secure resources. Only Black women used illegalities and instrumental relationships. I would argue that results from each strategy reflect how Black women invented responses, some innovative and some not, to external events that made life on welfare more difficult. In addition, what Black women did to take care of themselves and their families seemed based on the fact that they were faced with obstacles more often than women of other racial groups. For example, Black women reported they found it more difficult to secure housing than other women and tended to use speech acts as a way to ensure being housed. They were also more likely to be sanctioned

TABLE 2. Strategies Used to Address Economic Violence by Race/Ethnicity

Strategy	Race	Economic Violence Frequency (% of ethnic group)	TOTAL
Speech Acts	Black	7 (54%)	9
	White	2 (50%)	
	Latina	n/a	
	Asian	n/a	
	Other	n/a	
Fictive Kin	Black	3 (23%)	5
	White	1 (25%)	
	Latina	1 (33%)	
	Asian	n/a	
	Other	n/a	
Illegalities	Black	4 (30%)	4
	White	n/a	
	Latina	n/a	
	Asian	n/a	
	Other	n/a	
Instrumental Relationships	Black	2 (15%)	2
	White	n/a	
	Latina	n/a	
	Asian	n/a	
	Other	n/a	

and used instrumental friendships to ensure access to material resources such as food (Davis, 2006).

Intersection of Strategies to Address Violence and Poverty

In this section, I present women's responses to the overlapping spheres in which welfare reform policy shaped their needs during and after shelter stay (see Table 3). In discussing these survival strategies, it is important to keep in mind that these strategies are all in response to IPV and poverty, and some strategies addressed both while others addressed poverty alone. The strategies that these battered women used to deal with poverty were often extensions of those previously documented with different samples (e.g., Brownell, 2007; Hoff, 1990).

Case Study # 1 Solange: Speech Acts

Words are a forceful mediator for people living on the margins of society (Desjarlais, 1997), and battered women on welfare told stories in

TABLE 3. Types of Non-Violent Responses to IPV and to Poverty

Responses to Poverty	Responses to IPV	Responses to Poverty/IPV
Speech Acts		
Fictive Kin Networks	Kin Networks ◀──▶	Kin Networks
Instrumental Relations	Instrumental Relations ◀──▶	Instrumental Relations
Illegalities		

an attempt to offer a subjective perspective to their situation. These confessionals are often intended to manage the stigma of being on welfare and being perceived as fraudulent. Confessions are one way of coping with poverty as well as structural impediments that predictably deepened women's actual and perceived fears of poverty. Women also used speech acts to persuade people to help them, because talking had a purpose. In essence, women calculated what they might get in return for telling their story or revealing something about themselves. Sociolinguists distinguish between what is known as ordinary and institutional conversation (e.g., Drew & Heritage, 1992; Labov, 1972), although debates about dichotomizing conversation in this way suggest some limitations (McElhinny, 1997). Ordinary conversation involves non-standard speech patterns and familiar talk, similar to the way one might speak to a friend. Institutional conversation, on the other hand, is often characterized by "core goals, task orientation, and constraints" on what participants can say (p. 110), such as the way one might speak to Social Service personnel.

Women often switched to conversational style, utilizing ordinary conversation in institutional settings. Further, what they chose to talk about with agency staff was more personal than one might expect. In these cases, the women's audience was most often Social Service workers and housing/rental personnel. Women tried to convince Social Service caseworkers that aspects of welfare reform were contradictory to their own values (e.g., restrictions in attending college), hoping to prove they were worthy of the assistance they received.

The context of talking emerged from the dire circumstances in which women found themselves. Their disclosures, however, were not a reflection of democratic speech situations but rather were compelled by the need to survive and express the nature of power differentials between the speech "actor" and the listener. When women used speech acts with realtors, caseworkers, and employers, they often found themselves in unequal relations of power where the listener judged their worthiness. These relationships were entered into in part because welfare reform exacerbates the subordinate position from which poor battered women must operate in order to get what they need. Women often "confess" because they have to, not because they want to, and sometimes self-exposure is humiliating.

However, the speech acts in which mostly Black women engaged show that desperation often produced the use of more familiar, ordinary talk and confessions in institutional spaces instead of self-censure. We see the interplay of these two types of speech patterns in Solange's case. Solange needed to find a place to live, and her desperation lay in not wanting to return to her husband. She refused to live through her husband's "sickness" again (e.g., lining toothpicks up against the front door to determine if she had left the house when he was not home). She was determined to find housing, but was having difficulty.

Solange, age 37, was a former foster child who had survived childhood sexual abuse for many years. According to Solange, the secret of childhood sexual abuse festered into bulimia. Since no one believed her as a child, she found she was able to elicit a sympathetic response from institutional personnel through disclosure, not of her sexual assault but of her bulimia:

> My bulimia gives me a sense of control. I don't stick my finger down my throat like the others do. I just cough until my food comes up. But I've got it under control now. But I know when it's coming; it happens when I get anxious.

Solange used the confessional in an attempt to secure housing so she would not have to go back to her husband. Her quest for housing was often futile, perhaps due to the hidden hand of racializing. But she had a comeback to those who told her "we have nothing available." She confessed that she had bulimia. She would hold her chest, begin coughing, and with shortened breath, proclaim "my bulimia is coming on." It is important to note that Solange's preferred rental arrangement was Section VIII. She was unwilling, and for good reason, to accept housing assistance from Social Services because she did not want to live in a "slum," as she put it. She went to the Laneville Section VIII office and was told that nothing was available. Solange performed the bulimia "script," and to appease Solange the secretary immediately told her to fill out an application. This gesture had the effect of stabilizing

Solange's on-coming bulimic attack. On Solange's part, this was a creative but desperate attempt to capture control where she had none, to circumvent homelessness, and to establish a safe household for her and her daughters.

One housing administrator described the impact that women's speech acts had on her. She stated that when poor women came to her office, sat down, cried, and frequently told her every detail of their lives, she was moved: "Many of them tell their whole life story as a negotiating point to get a place to live." She admitted that she viewed women who told their stories a little differently than those who did not, and to the degree possible she tried to find housing for those women first.

Interviews with community advocates also revealed an increase in the use of speech acts as a survival strategy since the onset of welfare reform. Helen, an advocate who has been doing community work for 15 years, told me that welfare reform has caused women to really think through the kinds of arrangements they may need because of the crisis of benefit reduction, sanctioning, or case closure:

> They talk their landlords into letting them pay the rent in small portions. They say 'Next Monday, I'll give so and so amount.' They can't do this at the big complexes; they can only do it with private homeowners. Of course this limits women's choices for housing because they have to live in smaller buildings, like private homes, where they can negotiate with landlords. (Helen, community advocate)

Having no safe place to live was one of the biggest fears battered women faced, and talking one's way into or keeping an apartment made sense and sometimes worked. But sometimes Solange's speech acts were misdirected. For example, I know Solange thought I had some power to influence her entry into an apartment complex that was co-owned by Angel House and the River Valley Housing Authority. Twice, she told me how her condition could be neutralized if she knew she could get into the supportive housing program, coughing for the duration of the conversation. The routine of reminding those around her that her bulimia was triggered by anxiety was a different way of telling her story to bring about a positive outcome. She believed that if narrated and performed well enough to the right person, a deal might be struck, putting the odds of obtaining housing in her favor.

Gal (1991) points out that in sharing personal details about oneself, the listener judges your worthiness, which was precisely the women's intent. Women's verbal practices are an effort to represent their own experiences, and speech acts offer them the opportunity to provide a version of who they are and what their needs are. Simultaneously, by speaking up, they are contesting institutional inadequacies that have failed them, in this case the lack of safe and affordable housing. Successful responses to speech acts were found to motivate most women to continue using this strategy to help get their needs met. To whom they chose to disclose is as important as what they chose to disclose. Typically, they disclosed to formal institutional network personnel, such as Social Service caseworkers, housing authority staff, advocates, and employers. It was usually to someone they thought could offer immediate help and was rarely used in situations when women felt less certain of the outcome.

Case Study # 2 Clemmie: Creating Fictive Kin

Personal motivation is not usually sufficient to enable a woman to escape male violence. Hoff (1990) noted that battered women's survival of IPV incorporates the use of various forms of social networks. The use of networks may involve asking for, giving, receiving, or withholding help during a crisis around battering. A social network member is defined as anyone a battered woman can call on for help. Battered women use both formal and informal networks to help alleviate the crisis of IPV or to leave violent relationships. Sometimes institutional members are included in the network, but according to Dobash and Dobash (1979), not all interactions with institutional network members are positive. For example, police officers and other service workers often exacerbate a problem. Therefore, the use of calling the police or accessing social services as a strategy often occurs in times of crisis.

While women were only allowed to spend up to three months at the shelter, they came to know each other very well, and the relationships they developed lasted beyond shelter life. Because the escalation of violence in women's lives often severed family ties, women like Clemmie attempted to recreate the family that was lost due to violence. Clemmie is a 38-year old African American woman with four children. Her two oldest children are Shawnice, age 19 and Lena, 18. She also has two sons, James, age 15 and Henry, 9. Clemmie met a man whose abuse escalated over one year's time and included putting a gun in her mouth in front of her children. Because this man knew her social security number and had friends at social services, he was able to track her down and forced her to turn over to him all food stamps and cash assistance. This also meant he would know about any job she had in the future, so she was unable to work and therefore unable to meet the requirements of the PRWORA.

Clemmie's desire to reconstitute the family she missed while living at the shelter resulted in constructing a network of individuals who became her family and a source of income. Her network was composed of staff and shelter residents:

> Margaret, [a shelter advocate] is like a grandmother to my children. Josie [a resident] is like my daughter—'cause she's so close in age to Shawnice. Her daughter Shaneva is my granddaughter and I'm gonna teach her everything she needs to know about being Black—since her father is Black and she don't see him. Sheila is my sister. She's the person who makes me feel like a family. I know when she's sad and she trusts me. I miss my baby sister, so she's her for now. Alfonso, [a male advocate] is James and Henry's dad, and Sheila's son Marcel is like a younger brother to Henry because he needs someone to look up to him. Especially since he is so far away from his younger cousins.

Members of Clemmie's fictive kin were not only Black women from the shelter but also included White shelter staff as well as one other White woman, Josie. I would argue that the nature of need blurred the lines of race for Clemmie, because when it came to "making a family" to help through lean times, race and ethnic divisions seemed to be the least of her concerns.

Four months after arriving at the shelter in April of 1999, Clemmie received a budget of $450 toward her $500 rent, $104 in cash, and $171 in food stamps each month. She clearly needed more money because $171 did not cover food costs for the five people living in her household. Clemmie drew down from the $104 in cash she received. She used $50 to cover the difference of her rent and $54 for food, bringing her total food expenditure up to $225 a month. This translated into $45 per person or $1.50 per day for everyone. After those two expenses (rent and food), Clemmie had no money. To support her family she drew on her fictive kin network, some members of whom paid her to watch their children. The following excerpt from my field notes illustrates how Clemmie survived using the fictive kin network she created at the shelter.

The day I visited Clemmie's small apartment, it was full of people. Her daughter was lying across one of two old couches in the cramped living room watching television. Clemmie's niece was sitting on the other couch. Henry, Clemmie's son, told her that he wanted to go outside and ride his bike. In the middle of the room stood Josie, a former shelter resident holding Shaneva. Looking at me and pointing to Josie, she said, "Remember her, that's my daughter and that's my granddaughter." After the re-introduction, Josie turned to leave, and as she walked toward the door she handed Clemmie some money. Josie hugged Clemmie goodbye and left. After Josie's departure, Clemmie and I sat in the kitchen and talked during which time she revealed that her caseworker at Social Services recently threatened to cut her off financially because she was not working. I inquired about the money I saw Josie give her and Clemmie told me the details of how she made money baby sitting for women in her network:

> I need a little help. Sheila [her "sister"] gives me $60 a week for watching Marcel from 4 to 6:15 pm five days a week. But she's struggling, I know I could get more than that but I got to help my "sister" out. She can't give me any more. She gives me what she can give me. For Josie, [her "daughter"], I may watch the baby one day on the weekend; she'll bring me $20. I tell her no, but she insists. I also watch Linda's [another former resident] son. She has to work at the burger place 'cause DSS wouldn't give her anything. She works the midnight-to-eight shift, so he just sleeps over here. She pays me $50...I never thought about making a living doing the childcare thing. I used to make $11 something an hour working construction. But now, how I'm gonna live off of $52 every two weeks? What's that gonna do? Anything that keeps money coming in, that's regular, I'll do it.

Clemmie earned $130 a week from her babysitting jobs. The fictive kin network established months before while living at the shelter contributed to her ability to sustain her family. She, like other women cross-culturally, drew on a network to compensate for privation. From Jamaica to South Africa, the strategy of kin-network support has been substantively documented among women. Harrison (1997) showed that poor women in Jamaica living in urban areas have utilized networks to keep afloat as a result of structural adjustment programs that have reduced spending on social service needs for citizens. In another example, women's kinship relations in Tshunyane, South Africa (Donaldson, 1997) helped to negotiate and secure healthcare, a service hampered under the pressures of apartheid. Family networks and patterns of exchange have been widely discussed as a mechanism for accessing material resources, services, and information, which can influence family members' standards of living (Mencher, 1993).

Elaborating on the importance of networks, the creation of fictive kin networks in resource attainment transcends blood ties, similar to the findings from Stack's (1974) classic work on poor Blacks living in the Midwestern U.S. Fictive kinships work to smooth the interruption of public assistance benefits, sanctions, benefit reductions, and non-payment of benefits. These networks help unemployed women as well as those who were employed but lacked affordable resources such as child care. The vagaries of uncertainty caused by dislocation due to IPV as well as policies that penalize poor women were resolved in large measure through exchanges between network members. Women's survival depended on these networks, and they were aware of the responsibility that came with being integrated into one. One caution, of course, is that although networks are connected to a sense of obligation, they can and do expand and contract. The threads of kin or fictive-kin based networks can be stretched quite thin, especially when women have a limited number of people in their fictive kin circle.

Case Study #3 Sherita: Instrumental Friendships

Some women found themselves in the position of having to develop instrumental friendships, intentionally entering into functional relationships with both small business owners and sometimes with institutionally-affiliated individuals. These were people from whom the women could get something they needed. Relationships were constructed most often by women that had not developed fictive kin relations with other women while at the shelter. Landlords with one or two rental properties, grocery-store owners, and bus drivers were examples of non-institutionally affiliated individuals with whom women formed alliances. Women initiated the relationship by performing a "favor" for a person, and then banking that favor as a form of credit toward a future need. Beth, a White woman in her 40s who works with battered women, shared with me her observations about how instrumental relationships operate in the case of landlords:

> They find ways to be a good tenant. They will make sure that everything is clean, or quiet or something to please their landlords, so he/she will like them and give them slack. One woman had a small clerical job [along with receiving TANF funds]. She made friends

with the landlord up front and he liked her. She was conscientious about keeping her apartment and the rest of the building clean. She was very careful. And then when she had to have her car repaired, she knew she wouldn't also be able to pay her rent on time, but she was able to negotiate with the landlord [because of the favors she had done]. I know that the landlord applied for and got that apartment registered to accept Section VIII subsidies. The rules for Section VIII include timely payment of rent. With that, she should have been paying her rent on time but the landlord let her keep the arrangement of paying when she could. I just don't know how long these things will last. (Beth, battered women's advocate)

After moving into their apartments, many women took on the role of maintenance person or groundskeeper. For example, if the hallway light bulb blew out, they would purchase a replacement after drawing from their own limited resources. Or, without being asked, they would organize the garbage for pick-up, making sure that the recycled garbage was in the correct bags or placing other tenants' garbage in the appropriate place. Occasionally, women planted flowers or tended the landlord's garden. They did these things with no expectation of payment and the landlords never, to my knowledge, offered to repay them. Most women lived in owner-occupied units or houses, and many took on some building maintenance work knowing that there was no accounting for what they "spent," but in the end they expected something in return. They were building up moral credit with landlords and others, looking good in the eyes of people they did not know intimately but from whom they could request a favor at some point. For example, Sherita, described earlier, prepared meals for the owner of a small grocery store, and expected that she could "buy" food using the moral credit when her food stamps were reduced or eliminated. She also invited the program director of Catholic Charities to her house for dinner. Her rationale was that cultivating personal relationships with service providers would facilitate securing basic needs if her benefits were reduced. Sherita, like other women, lived by the art of making arrangements (Pardo, 1996), and her instrumental friendships were organized in terms of how deficits could be managed (Wolf, 1966). This was a necessary strategy in light of how often women were sanctioned, experienced benefit reductions, or could not make ends meet no matter how hard they tried.

In its practicality, instrumental friendships draw on the burden of emotion that accrues from an exchange of mutual assistance, but these engagements are tenuous for several reasons. First, if a woman does not provide a favor, the alliance is not initiated. Second, the friendship does not exist between equals because the woman is in a subordinate position and risks being exploited. As Wolf (1966) states, "the relation contains an element which provides sanctions internal to the relation itself" (p. 13). Further, the relationship does not change a woman's status from being poor. Clearly, alliances were developed in the hope that the person or "donor" would have enough sympathy to assist them when it became necessary.

Offers of assistance on the part of the donor were more substantial than simply doing a favor. Aid offered by the donor was crucial to women's survival because without it, women might go hungry or lose their apartments. As noted earlier, relationships of this type developed out of need mostly because women's support networks were thin or non-existent.

Case Study #4 Elizabeth: Illegalities

According to Richie (1996), abuse is recognized as a factor in women's aggressive behavior and engagement in illegal activities. Richie argues that none of the five women she studied had committed violent crimes before abuse from intimate partners. Abuse was a major factor, however, in women's aggression toward the men who threatened them. The paths to illegal behavior reveal a continuity of messages about taking care of oneself, incorporated into adult consciousness after being battered. The women ultimately felt that the best way to resolve their problems was to take care of their own business.

However, none of the women in my study reported any illegal behavior for which they were arrested, using the term "illegal" to loosely encompass things women were willing to do that fell outside of "acceptable" and "normative" female behavior as well as in a strict legal sense. The point here is the conceptual link between behavioral acts not condoned by societal/institutional standards or legalities, and limited options battered women possess. Among women in Richie's study, illegal activity was seen as a response to violence. The women in my study also used forms of illegality in response to the combination of violence and poverty in order to avoid returning to a violent household.

Elizabeth, a Black woman in her 30s, was born in the West Indies and raised in Great Britain. Her family, consisting of her mother, father, and five siblings, came to live in New York when she was six years old. Elizabeth was intellectually gifted and received a full scholarship to attend a prestigious private high school, followed by attendance at an Ivy League university on the East Coast. Elizabeth had two children, Kamari, age 5 and Olu, age 3, by her husband John, who was a disabled veteran. Kamari had severe eczema and a learning disability, and Olu had severe asthma. The two boys were her pride and joy. "Every breath I take," she told me, is toward ensuring that their lives were stabilized. She received public assistance in light of her husband's abuse and after becoming unemployed. She told me, "I had lost my job. I didn't have money and my unemployment had not kicked in. We had no food...I went on social services."

We sat down in the television room at the shelter one afternoon. She told me that her husband had been awarded court-ordered visitation rights and had seen his sons somewhat regularly over the past three years since their separation. Elizabeth tried to include John in decisions about their children, especially the oldest (Kamari) who was having difficulty in school. One evening she took Olu with her when she went to speak with John about some issues Kamari was having at school. John started yelling at her and blaming her for Kamari's problems. His rage turned physical and he picked Elizabeth up in front of Olu and held her against the wall by her neck. Choking, she said, she begged him to stop and finally wrangled free from his grip. She and Olu ran out of the house into a cab that happened to be cruising by.

Knowing that this would trigger a flight response on Elizabeth's part, John called her later that night threatening to "get her" if she took the children someplace where he could not see them. Of course, she was concerned about what he might do to her, and Elizabeth came to Angel House. Elizabeth arrived at Angel House with an open Social Services case from another city where she had Section VIII housing. She tried to use it in Laneville. However, a community worker explained to me that River Valley County did all it could to prevent women from other parts of the state from receiving benefits within the county. Unable to locate a place to live that would be safe for her children, Elizabeth shared with me that she had considered moving out of state in spite of the fact that the children's father threatened to have her arrested:

> I don't think I have a choice. I think making enough money to buy a plane ticket to Great Britain is what I might have to do. The children don't have dual citizenship, but I do. As soon as I hit British soil, there will be a support system, not like here.

After three months of trying to establish a household in Laneville, Elizabeth decided to move to Michigan, an area of the country where she felt she could be comfortable and could pursue work. In so doing, she was acting illegally in violation of the court-mandated visitation order handed down on behalf of her husband. In spite of the fact that the boys' father had threatened to have her arrested, she decided that she would "rather be a fugitive." Elizabeth's decision to be a fugitive not only arose from wanting to get away from her husband, but also "to get away from the eyes of the system." In order to get the services she needed to rebuild her life, she would once again have to tell the story of her abuse. However, Elizabeth was unconvinced that the system was effective enough to warrant such self-exposure yet again.

One goal of welfare reform was to reduce the number of people receiving assistance, yet it seemed that bureaucratic ineffectiveness prevented Elizabeth from becoming self-sufficient. This was not so much a situation in which a woman was mandated to meet unreasonable demands as it was a situation where "holding the line" was played out with Elizabeth. Of course, diversionary tactics that deeply frustrate people so that they want to end the Department of Social Service application process is quite effective for roll reduction.

Among the women in this ethnographic study, desperation and violence forced them to make strategic choices in order to survive. There are a limited number of choices that battered women in poverty can make (Purvin, 2003). Some battered women return to former batterers to ensure economic solvency, yet none of the women I spoke with entered into serial relationships during the time that I knew them, and I was aware of only one woman who returned to her batterer. However, women did sustain contact with former batterers mostly for childcare reasons, a connection precipitated by sanctions, court orders, and work mandates.

In the absence of court-ordered visitation, women often recruited a former batterer, who was generally the father of their children, to provide childcare services. This was sometimes an illegal act that could result in losing their children to state child service agencies or being charged with child endangerment due to "failure to protect." Nevertheless, several women made these arrangements in order to attend mandatory training programs or work. Women would then promise their batterer they would not ask for child support, because in their view providing childcare was an "even exchange" for child support.

DISCUSSION

Violence and Welfare Use

Documenting the lack of economic resources in battered women's decision-making processes has been a critical finding in research on

IPV against women with regard to leaving and remaining away from battering relationships. As can be seen above, the stories of women who were victims of IPV show how strategies to overcome poverty shape women's choices.

Gondolf (1988), for example, studied the shelter exit plans of 800 women in Texas and found that access to an independent income were primary considerations. Raphael (1995) found that most shelter residents use welfare to end the violence in their lives. However, PRWORA shredded the historical safety net that provided poor women with guaranteed assistance. As mentioned earlier, Aid to Families with Dependent Children (AFDC, also dubbed TANF) became a temporary program that was time limited to five years. Further, in order to receive assistance, a work-first policy was mandated. The implications of this policy is that all recipients must be directed toward subsidized or unsubsidized employment, work training programs, or any set of activities that would ultimately lead to work as a requirement for receiving assistance. Failure to comply with the work mandates, or as is often the case, administrative error, results in being sanctioned (i.e., elimination of benefits for a period of time) or case closure, placing recipients at high risk for catastrophic poverty (Davis et al., 2003).

Ending benefits obviously jeopardizes a poor women's ability to escape abusive partners. Aware that battered women use welfare to address the violence in their lives, battered women's advocates challenged welfare reform on several fronts, stating that patterns of violence would interfere with women's employment or engagement in work-related activities. As in the present sample, several other researchers have shown that women's abusive partners sabotage women's efforts toward economic independence by injuring them and/or preventing them from successfully meeting work or work-related activity requirements (Raphael & Tolman 1997; Washington State Institute for Public Policy, 1993).

Results from a Massachusetts study of 734 women receiving welfare in 40 of the state's 42 welfare offices found that 64.9% of women had experienced some form of physical violence in their lives, and 19.5% had reported such abuse in the past year (Allard, Albelda, Colten, & Cosenza, 1997). A Salt Lake City study of 3,147 domestic violence incidents found that 38% to 41% of the women had opened welfare cases within one year either before or after the incident. The short length of time between reporting the incident and opening a welfare case suggests a connection between domestic violence and welfare use, where welfare is often used as way to gain independence (Brandwein, 1999a). Lack of resources is seen as a factor that may force women to stay with or return to their batterers. Indeed, welfare reform may be viewed as a form of structural violence that can be interpreted as revictimization in the non-intimate sphere, due to the possibility of sanctions, low-income employment, and lack of job protection that compromise women's ability to create the economically autonomous lives they need to keep away from violent partners (Susser, 1998).

It is important to examine violence, poverty, and welfare reform policy in relation to market-place forces, especially because globalization and deindustrialization have reduced the ability of poor people to earn a living wage in many communities across the country (Goode & Maskovsky, 2002). The site of the present ethnographic research, River Valley County in New York state, had economic circumstances that mimic those of other communities across the U.S. The county experienced precipitous decreases in major manufacturing industries and rises in technology and service sectors. In response, local governments have attempted to contain economic erosion while simultaneously devising revitalization schemes. At the intersection of these phenomena are poor and working class people receiving public assistance for whom economic security is uncertain and often unattainable. For battered women, the problems are obviously exacerbated.

Let me restate how important it is to uncover the effects of welfare reform on abused women in light of evidence that male abusers undermine their efforts to leave the relationship and achieve economic autonomy. In this context, the violence/poverty interface takes on increasingly complicated contours. Poverty, as one circumstance of violence, clearly influences battered women's life choices. Because social violence may be understood on a continuum where economic fragility and women's differential access to resources often force them into the welfare system, so too must battered women's responses to IPV be understood within such contexts. The case studies used above clearly illustrate the strategies and patterns of response that battered women may use to deal with both a lack of economic resources and lack of interpersonal safety they face every day. In the face of these pressures, it may not be surprising that women choose to respond with violence against their batterers. Clearly, however, the present ethnographic study shows they often find other ways to address the violence in their lives.

NOTES

1. Mandatory arrest laws provided police with the charge to make an arrest under specific circumstances as an effective measure to protect women (see O'Dell, this issue).
2. All names used in this article are fictitious for reasons of confidentiality.
3. The Family Violence Amendment to the Personal Responsibility and Work Opportunity Reconciliation Act [Sec. 402(a) (7)] permits states to screen for domestic violence for candidates applying for assistance and those being dropped from assistance programs, and refers domestic violence victims to counseling and determines if certain welfare requirements should be waived (see Kurz, 1999).

REFERENCES

Allard, M. A., Albelda, R., Colten, M. E., & Cosenza, C. (1997). *In harm's way? Domestic violence, AFDC receipt, and welfare reform in Massachusetts.* Boston, MA: McCormack Institute.

Anglin, M. (1998). Feminist perspectives on structural violence. *Identities 5*(2), 145-151.

Archer, J. (1999). Assessment of the reliability of the Conflict Tactics Scale: A meta-analytic review. *Journal of Interpersonal Violence, 14,* 1263-1289.

Bohannon, J. R., Dosser, D. A., & Lindley, S. E. (1995). Using couple data to determine domestic violence rates: An attempt to replicate previous work. *Violence and Victims, 10,* 133-141.

Brandwein, R. A. (1999a). Family violence and welfare use: A report from the field. In R. A. Brandwein (Ed.), *Battered women, children and welfare reform: The ties that bind* (pp. 45-57). Thousand Oaks, CA: Sage

Brandwein, R. A. (Ed.) (1999b). *Battered women, children, and welfare reform: The ties that bind.* Thousand Oaks, CA: Sage

Browne, A, & Bassuk, S. (1997). Intimate violence in the lives of homeless and poor housed women: Prevalence and patterns in an ethnically diverse sample. *American Journal of Orthopsychiatry, 6,* 261-278.

Browne, A., Salomon, A., & Bassuk, S. (1999). Impact of partner violence on poor women's capacity to maintain work. *Violence Against Women, 5*(4), 393-426.

Brownell, P. (2007). Women, welfare, work, and domestic violence. In A. R. Roberts (Ed.), *Battered women and their families* (pp. 291-311). New York, NY: Springer.

Clifford, J. O. (1999, November 24). *Domestic case arrests of women rise.* Retrieved May 4, 2004, Associated Press Writer location, http://www.menweb.org/batapwmn.html.

Cook, S. L. (2002). Self-reports of sexual, physical and nonphysical abuse perpetration: A comparison of three measures. *Violence Against Women, 8*(5), 541-565.

Davies, J., Lyon, E., & Monti-Catania, D. (1998). *Safety planning with battered women: Complex lives, difficult choices.* Thousand Oaks, CA: Sage.

Davis, D. A. (2006). *Between a rock and a hard place: Battered Black women and welfare reform.* Albany, NY: State University of New York Press.

Davis, D. A., Aparicio, A., Jacobs, A., Kochiyama, A., Mullings, L., Queeley, A., et al. (2003). Working it off: Welfare reform, workfare and work experience programs in New York City. *Souls: A Critical Journal of Black Politics, Culture, and Society, 5*(2), 22-41.

Desjarlais, R. (1997). *Shelter blues: Sanity and selfhood among the homeless.* Philadelphia, PA: Pennsylvania University Press.

Dobash, R. E., & Dobash, R. P. (1979). *Violence against wives*. New York: Free Press.

Donaldson, D. R. (1997). Our women keep our skies from falling: Women's networks and survival imperatives in Tshunyane, South Africa. In G. Mikell (Ed.), *African feminism: The politics of survival in Sub-Saharan Africa* (pp. 257-275). Philadelphia, PA: University of Pennsylvania Press.

Drew, P., & Heritage, J. (Eds.) (1992). *Talk at work: Interaction in institutional settings*. Cambridge: Cambridge University Press.

Gal, S. (1991). Between speech and silence: The problematics of research on language and gender. In M. diLeonardo (Ed.), *Gender at the crossroads of knowledge* (pp. 175-203). Berkeley, CA: University of California Press.

Galtung, J. (1969). Violence, peace, and peace research. *Journal of Peace Research, 6*, 170-171.

Goldberg, C. (1999, November 23). Spouse abuse crackdown, surprisingly, nets many women. *New York Times*, Section A, p. 16.

Gondolf, E. (1988). *Battered women as survivors: An alternative to treating learned helplessness*. Lexington, MA: Lexington.

Goode, J., & Maskovsky, J. (Eds.) (2002). *The new poverty studies: The ethnography of power, politics, and impoverished peoples in the United States*. New York: New York University Press.

Harrison, F. V. (1997). The gendered politics and violence of structural adjustments: A view from Jamaica. In L. Lamphere, H. Ragone, & P. Zavella (Eds.), *Situated lives: Gender and culture in everyday life* (pp. 451-468). New York: Routledge.

Hearn, M. E. (2000). *Dangerous indifference: New York City's failure to implement the family violence option*. New York: NOW Legal Defense and Education Fund for Women.

Hoff, L. A. (1990). *Battered women as survivors*. New York: Routledge.

Housing Opportunity Program Extension Act of 1996, Pub. L. 104-120, 110 Stat. 834.

Johnson, M. P., & Ferraro, K. J. (2000). Research on domestic violence in the 1990s: Making distinctions. *Journal of Marriage and the Family, 62*, 948-963.

Kurz, D. (1999). Women, welfare and domestic violence. In G. Mink (Ed.), *Whose welfare?* (pp. 132-151). Ithaca, NY: Cornell University Press.

Labov, W. (1972). *Language in the inner city*. Philadelphia, PA: University of Pennsylvania Press.

Leisring, P. A., Dowd, L., & Rosenbaum, A. (2003). Treatment of partner aggressive women. *Journal of Aggression, Maltreatment & Trauma, 7*(1/2), 257 - 276.

Lyon, E. (2000). *Welfare poverty and abused women: New research and its implications*. Harrisburg, PA: National Resource Center on Domestic Violence.

Malloy, K. A., McCloskey, K. A., Grigsby, N., & Gardner, D. (2003). Women's use of violence within intimate relationships. *Journal of Aggression, Maltreatment & Trauma, 6*(2), 37-59.

Martin, M. E. (1997). Double your trouble: Dual arrest in family violence. *Journal of Family Violence, 12*, 139-157.

McElhinny, B. (1997). Ideologies of public and private language in sociolinguistics. In R. Wodak (Ed.), *Gender and discourse* (pp. 106-139). Thousands Oaks, CA: Sage.

Mencher, J. P. (1993). Female-headed female-supported households in India: Who are they and what are their survival strategies? In J. P. Mencher & A. Okongwu (Eds.), *Where did all the men go? Female headed, female-supported households in cross-cultural perspective* (pp. 203-232). Boulder, CO: Westview Press.

National Poverty Center. (n.d.). *Poverty in the United States: 2004 poverty thresholds, selected family types.* Retrieved May 20, 2007 from, http://www.npc.umich.edu/poverty/

NOW Legal Defense and Education Fund. (2004). *Reading between the lines: Women's poverty in the United States 2003.* New York. Retrieved January 10, 2005 from, http://www.legalmomentum.org/womeninpoverty.pdf

O'Dell, A. (2007). Why do police arrest victims of domestic violence? The need for comprehensive training and investigative protocols. *Journal of Aggression, Maltreatment & Trauma, 15*(3/4), 53-73.

O'Leary, K. D., Barling, J., Arias, I., Rosenbaum, A., Malone, J., & Tyree, A. (1989). Prevalence and stability of physical aggression between spouses: A longitudinal analysis. *Journal of Consulting and Clinical Psychology, 57,* 263-268.

O'Leary, K. D., Vivian, D., & Malone, J. (1992). Assessment of physical aggression against women in marriage: The need for a multimodal assessment. *Behavioral Assessment, 14,* 5-14.

Pardo, I. (1996). *Managing existence in Naples: Morality, action and structure.* Cambridge: Cambridge University Press.

Personal Responsibility and Work Opportunity Reconciliation Act of 1996, Pub.L. 104-193, 110 Stat. 2105.

Purvin, D. M. (2003). Weaving a tangled safety net: The intergenerational legacy of domestic violence and poverty. *Violence Against Women, 9,* 1263-1277.

Raphael, J. (1995). Domestic violence and welfare receipt: The unexplored barrier to employment. *Georgetown Journal on Fighting Poverty, 3,* 29-34.

Raphael, J. (1999). The family violence option: An early assessment. *Violence Against Women, 5*(4), 449-466.

Raphael, J., & Tolman, R. (1997). *Trapped by poverty/trapped by abuse: New evidence documenting the relationship between domestic violence and welfare.* Project for Research on Welfare, Work and Domestic Violence: Taylor Institute & University of Michigan Press.

Rennison C. M., & Welchans, S. (2000). *Intimate partner violence.* Washington, DC: Bureau of Justice Statistics. NCJ 178247.

Renzetti, C. (2001). One strike and you're out: Implications of a federal crime control policy for battered women. *Violence Against Women, 7*(6), 685-698.

Richie, B. E. (1996). *Compelled to crime: The gender entrapment of battered black women.* New York & London: Routledge.

Saltzman, L. E., Fanslow J. L., McMahon P. M, & Shelley, G. A. (1999). *Intimate partner violence surveillance: Uniform definitions and recommended data elements.* Atlanta, GA: National Center for Injury Prevention and Control.

Sheffield, R. (1995, May 30). State law offers help for battered women. *Standard-Times.* Retrieved May 15, 2004 from, http://www.s-t.com/projects/DomVio/statelaw.HTML

Stack. C. (1974). *All our kin: Strategies for survival in a black community.* New York: Harper & Row.

Stark, E., & Flitcraft, A. (1988). Violence among intimates: An epidemiological review. In V. Van Hasselet, R. Morrison, A. Bellack, & M. Hersen (Eds.), *Handbook of family violence* (pp. 293-297). New York: Plenum.

Straus, M. A. (1999). The controversy over domestic violence by women: A methodological, theoretical, and sociology of science analysis. In X. B. Arriaga & S. Oskamp (Eds.), *Violence in intimate relationships* (pp. 17-44). Thousand Oaks, CA: Sage.

Strauss, M. A., & Gelles, R. J. (1986). Societal change and change in family violence from 1975 to 1985 as revealed by two national surveys. *Journal of Marriage and the Family, 48,* 465-479.

Susser, I. (1996). The construction of poverty and homeless in U.S. cities. *Annual Review of Anthropology, 25,* 411-435.

Susser, I. (1998). Inequality, violence, and gender relations in a global city: New York, 1986-1996. *Identities, 5*(2), 219-247.

Swan, S., & Snow, D. L. (2002). A typology of women's use of violence in intimate relationships. *Violence Against Women, 8*(3), 286-319.

U.S. Department of Health and Human Services. (2004). *Women's health USA 2004.* Rockville, MD: Author. Retrieved January 19, 2005 from, http://www.mchb.hrsa.gov/whusa04/index.htm#toc

U.S. Department of Housing and Urban Development. (1997). *Implementation of the "one strike" policy.* Washington DC: Author.

Washington State Institute for Public Policy. (1993). *Over half of women on public assistance in Washington State reported physical or sexual abuse as adults.* Olympia, WA: Author.

Websdale, N. (1998). *Rural woman battering and the justice system: An ethnography.* Thousand Oaks, CA: Sage.

Wolf, E. R. (1966). Kinship, friendship, and patron-client relations in complex societies. In M. Banton (Ed.), *The social anthropology of complex societies* (pp. 1-22). London, UK: Tavistock Publications.

Worden, R. E., & Pollitz, A. (1984). Police arrests in domestic disturbances: A further look. *Law and Society Review, 18*(1), 105-119.

Submitted: May 5, 2005
Revised: May 29, 2005
Revised: May 29, 2007
Accepted: May 29, 2007

Using the Theory of Gender and Power to Examine Experiences of Partner Violence, Sexual Negotiation, and Risk of HIV/AIDS Among Economically DisadvantagedWomen in Southern India

Subadra Panchanadeswaran, PhD, MSW
Sethulakshmi C. Johnson, CMSC
Vivian F. Go, PhD, MPH
A. K. Srikrishnan, BA
Sudha Sivaram, DrPh
Suniti Solomon, MD
Margaret E. Bentley, PhD
David Celentano, MHS, ScD

Although men contracting the human immunodeficiency virus (HIV) worldwide outnumbered women early in the epidemic, women have gradually become equal in infection rates. In 1998, women constituted 41% of the people affected by HIV globally, but by 2004, nearly 50% of people globally living with HIV are women (UNAIDS, 2004). Feminization of this disease underscores the importance of including women in HIV and acquired immune deficiency syndrome (AIDS) prevention efforts. Unprotected heterosexual contact is one of the primary causes of the spread of sexually transmitted infections and HIV/AIDS. In countries around the world, women's low social status and high economic dependency on men heightens women's vulnerability to infections due to constraints in condom negotiation, discussing sexual norms and expectations with their partners, and limited options for leaving risky and sometimes violent relationships (Heise, 1993; Rao Gupta, 2002). Research evidence points to the intersections of HIV and intimate partner violence, suggesting that HIV infection may be a risk factor for and potential consequence of violence against women (Dunkle et al., 2004; El Bassel et al., 1998; Maman, Campbell, Sweat, & Gielan, 2002; Martin & Curtis, 2004; McDonnell, Gielen, & O'Campo, 2003; Wingood & DiClemente, 1997). Violence may increase women's risk for HIV/AIDS through the following mechanisms: (a) women in violent relationships may be afraid or unable to negotiate condom use (Davila, 2000, 2002; El-Bassel, Gilbert, Rajah, Foleno, & Frye, 2000; Koenig et al., 2003, 2004); and (b) women who have experienced violence in the past may be more likely to engage in HIV high-risk behaviors (Jinich, Paul, & Stall, 1998; Lodico & DiClemente, 1994; Wingood & DiClemente, 1997).

Outside of Africa, India has the largest number of people living with HIV (UNAIDS, 2004), with over 5.1 million infected individuals (National AIDS Control Organization [NACO], 2004). While HIV rates among women in the general population in India are low (Celentano et al., 2001), recent research has pointed to the spread of infection among married, monogamous women (Gangakhedkar, et al., 1997; Newmann et al., 2000). Indian women's vulnerability is increased as a result of inequitable social structures based on gender (Majumdar, 2004), male resistance to condom use (World Health Organization [WHO], 2000), and higher prevalence of risky sexual behaviors among men (Martin et al., 1999).

Current AIDS prevention strategies often promote the reduction in number of sexual partners, increased condom use, and prompt and appropriate treatment of sexually transmitted infections (Heise & Elias, 1995). However, these strategies do not address the socio-cultural realities and complexities of sexual decision making (Taylor, 1995) for many women that have been highlighted by research, including non-consensual sex, fear of partner violence, loss of livelihood/economic support, and inability to effectively and consistently negotiate condom use to prevent infections (Rao Gupta & Weiss, 1993).

A Theoretical Framework to Examine Women's Vulnerability to HIV/AIDS

Robert Connell (1987) developed an integrated Theory of Gender and Power that focused on three fundamental intertwined structures, namely: (a) sexual division of labor, (b) sexual division of power, and (c) the structure of cathexis (affective attachments and social norms). According to this theory, these three structures are present at both the societal and institutional levels, and social mechanisms play an active role in maintaining them. This results in gender inequities in all spheres of women's lives, including domestic, economic, and socio-cultural dimensions. The interactions between all of these elements produce gender disparities and inequities that serve to heighten women's vulnerability in various spheres, including women's health (Connell).

Wingood and DiClemente (2000) extended Connell's theory to develop a public health model that highlighted the various contextual and biological risk factors that affect women's risk for HIV/AIDS (see Figure 1). These authors used past research to identify specific exposures and risks that heighten women's vulnerability to HIV. This paper will use Wingood and DiClemente's model to shed light on poor, urban women from slums of southern India and their vulnerability to HIV/AIDS. The Theory of Gender and Power will be used to examine the data across the three dimensions of economic constraints, power disparities, and cultural norms. However, due to limited data availability, only selected dimensions of Wingood and DiClemente's model will be examined in this paper. From the structure of sexual division of labor, only poverty and high demand/low control work environments will be examined. Specific focus will be on the physical exposures of sexual division of power, such as partner violence and client violence (in the case of sex workers), women's experiences of male resistance to engage in safe sex despite high risk behaviors, risks posed by alcohol use, inabilities to successfully assert themselves and negotiate condom use, and perceived lack of control in intimate relationships. Women's entrapment in inequitable cultural norms will be examined in the structure of cathexis. Finally, strategies used by some women to resist unwanted sex will also be highlighted. It should be noted that biological exposures/risk factors will not be addressed.

FIGURE 1. Theory of gender and power: Women's exposure and risk for HIV (model adapted from categories given by Wingood and DiClemente, 2000). *Aspects of the model addressed in the current paper.

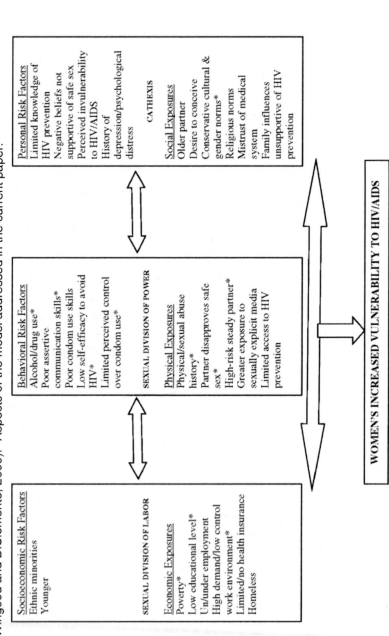

WINGOOD AND DICLEMENTE'S ADAPTATION
OF THE THEORY OF GENDER AND POWER
AND WOMEN'S VULNERABILITY TO HIV

Sexual Division of Labor

Across cultures, women and men have been socialized to engage in gender-specific occupations. The structure of sexual division of labor highlights the gendered nature of work that accords men relatively higher participation, status, and remuneration in the workplace as compared to women. The resulting economic imbalance may force women to be financially dependent on men, thereby creating vulnerability in all spheres (Wingood & DiClemente, 2000). Economic dependence on partners constrains women to sacrifice adoption of health-protective behaviors, including overlooking partner infidelities as well as violent behavior (Gupta, Weiss, & Whelan, 1995). Additionally, social mechanisms ensure an almost exclusive women's presence in "unpaid nurturing work" (Wingood & DiClemente, p. 542) such as child care, care of the sick and elderly, housework, and domestic work. This perpetuates disparities not only in income, but also in social status. Gendered division of labor ensures women's lack or limited access to economic, educational, and other resources, which may in turn produce adverse health outcomes. Commerical sex work is an example of the economic exposure in this structure that highlights 'high demand/low control' work environments for women that heightens their vulnerability in multiple ways. While the pathways leading women into the sex trade are varied and complex, poverty is one of the main factors that force many women to accept sex work as the only means of earning a livelihood for themselves and their children. Nevertheless, it is also an industry that perpetuates severe sexual exploitation of women at the cost of safer sex in which the industry entrepreneurs stand to gain (Adkins, 1995 as cited in Wingood & DiClemente).

In India's patriarchal society, which accords males the exclusive privilege to engage in sex outside marriage, commercial sex networks flourish (Venkataramana & Sarada, 2001). Majumdar (2004) found that circumstantial poverty and loss of the primary wage earner played a vital role in increasing women's vulnerability and eventual acceptance of sex work in India. A significant proportion of sex workers in Kerala, India were married, abused, deserted, stripped of property, and even sold into the sex trade by their husbands and hence accepted sex work as a means to earn a livelihood (Jayasree, 2004). Hence, in the context of

HIV prevention, it is important to recognize that when economic survival constitutes a top priority, sex workers' abilities to engage in negotiation may be irrelevant compared to their knowledge about condom
use and their abilities to negotiate with their clients (Santow, 1995). A
small proportion of sex workers in Mumbai, India requested that clients
use condoms, yet never turned away those who refused because it meant
loss of livelihood (Bhave et al., 1995).

Women's economic vulnerabilities as shown in the Sexual Division
of Labor approach formed the basis of our exploration in the current
study. We expected that female sex workers who typically work in
'high demand/low control' work environments, as well as poor women
from slums who lack financial and educational resources, would be
more vulnerable to HIV.

Sexual Division of Power

Power differentials between the sexes are a fundamental element of
gender and power theory (Connell, 1987). In addition to controlling financial assets, men exert power "through control, authority, and coercion within heterosexual relationships" (Raj, Silverman, Wingood, &
DiClemente, 1999, p. 276). Gender differentials in power manifest most
directly in the case of physical and sexual violence against women. Furthermore, power relations between the sexes are an important determi-
nant of the outcome of sexual negotiations (George, 1998; Go et al.,
2003; Santow, 1995).

Research has shown that accusations of a woman's infidelity are
common tactics used by male partners to force women into sexual relations (Davila, 2000; El-Bassel et al., 2000; George, 1998). In addition,
women's submission to non-consensual sex is often in response to
threats/use of physical violence (Holland & Ramazanoglu, 1992;
Ravindran & Balasubramanian, 2004). Fear of violence is an important
factor that impedes women from initiating condom negotiation with
their partners, especially since power imbalances have been shown to
be a major impediment in women's abilities to negotiate condom use
(Amaro, 1995; Heise, & Elias, 1995; Monahan, Miller, & Rothspan,
1997; Pulerwitz, Amaro, De Jong, & Gortmaker, 2002; Wingood &
DiClemente, 1998). Unfortunately, condom use is entirely male-con-
trolled. For instance, research evidence points to power differentials in
'female sex worker-male client' relationships where fear of violence
from clients deters women from initiating condom use (Asthana &
Oostvogels, 1996; Cusick, 1998; Sanders, 2004).

Another behavioral risk factor that accentuates power divisions is alcohol use, especially by male partners. Alcohol consumption has been strongly associated with coercive sex and heightened intimate partner violence by men (Koenig et al., 2003, 2004). In a study of pregnant women in an antenatal clinic in Pune city, India, 30% reported physical/mental abuse and/or alcohol/drug abuse by their partners (Shrotri et al., 2003). In a study among women and men in low-income communities in Mumbai, George (1998) found that for some women, forced sex was common when their male partners abused alcohol. Studies in the Philippines, Peru, Sri Lanka, and Guatemala (Heise & Elias, 1995), as well as studies conducted among Mexican-American women in the US (Davila, 2002), have shown similar results.

Wingood and DiClemente (2000) underscore women's low self-efficacy and confidence to negotiate condom use within abusive sexual relationships with men. The spread of HIV among married, monogamous women in India (Gangakhedkar et al., 1997; Newmann et al., 2000) points to their partners' high-risk behaviors as a clear manifestation of power differentials between genders. Male social power places women in vulnerable positions as a result of their inability to negotiate sexual behaviors.

In our study, we explored sex workers' and socio-economically disadvantaged women's vulnerability to HIV in the context of client/partner violence, alcohol use, male partner's high-risk behaviors, and women's perceptions of lack of control in their intimate relationships.

Cathexis

The structure of cathexis refers to societal norms and expectations regarding women's sexual behavior characterized by their sexual and emotional attachments to men (Wingood & DiClemente, 2000). According to this structure, gender inequities result from societal gender role prescriptions and socialization patterns. When women internalize and accept traditional and oppressive gender roles that impact behavior, this further erodes women's power in intimate relationships, which in turn affects their capacities to resist abuse (Raj et al., 1999). Cultural factors, such as the stigma of divorce and separation, were cited as key reasons that keep women in abusive relationships for prolonged periods in many qualitative studies (Acevedo, 2000; Hassouneh-Phillips, 2001; Rose, Campbell, & Kub, 2000). Go and colleagues (2003) found that although women and men implied that there was a level of acceptability regarding domestic violence, the level of acceptability varied by the justification of the violent act.

In the current study, we explored if higher degrees of acceptance of traditional gender norms would negatively influence women's abilities to control the outcomes of their efforts at sexual negotiation and therefore increase their vulnerability to HIV infection.

METHODS

Site

The findings for this paper are drawn from an on-going NIMH-funded randomized HIV prevention trial that examines the effectiveness of the use of Community Popular Opinion Leaders (CPOL) in disseminating HIV prevention messages in five countries: China, India, Peru, Russia, and Zimbabwe. Partners for the India site are Johns Hopkins University (Baltimore, MD) and the Y.R. Gaitonde Center for AIDS Research and Education (YRG-CARE), a non-profit, non-governmental organization based in Chennai city in the south-eastern Indian state of Tamil Nadu. Data were collected from residents in low-income communities. Typically, these communities lack adequate basic amenities and are designated as 'slums' by the Tamil Nadu Slum Clearance Board.

Sample and Data Collection

Qualitative data collection such as social mapping, participant observation, key informant interviews, and in-depth interviews were used to collect data. In the initial stages, project staff from YRG-CARE visited the slums regularly to identify key informants from various sites in the communities, explain study objectives, and enlist participation. The key informants were instrumental in helping to identify other potential participants by referring the staff to other members in the community. During discussions with informants, wine shops emerged as a possible venue to examine the context of HIV risk and hence a few wine shop patrons served as key informants and a "snow-ball" sampling technique was adopted to identify others in the social/sexual networks, including wine shop patrons, female sex workers, and male clients of sex workers. As part of the formative ethnography, trained female and male ethnographers conducted in-depth interviews with a total of 32 females and 38 males from the community. Interviewers were also trained to refer respondents to services whenever needed and also in instances where the interview content was upsetting for respondents.[1] Each participant completed two in-depth interviews, the first being a rapport-building interview and the second focusing on more sensitive topics such as sexual practices, sexual negotiation, and experiences of partner violence. Interviews were conducted in a private location and lasted about two hours. The informed consent forms and all other procedures were approved by the Institutional Review Boards from both Johns Hopkins University and YRG-CARE.

Data Analysis

Interviews were conducted in Tamil and subsequently transcribed and translated into English. Transcripts were randomly checked by the lead ethnographer and project manager at the site and also by a researcher (5th author) for accuracy of translation and representation of concepts. Data were analyzed using ATLAS.TI version 4.1 (Muhr, 1997). A broad coding plan was developed with HIV prevention themes in mind. Two researchers (3rd and 5th author) independently coded the interview transcripts and compared them for common themes. Finally, the first author used Wingood and DiClemente's (2000) adapted version of the Theory of Gender and Power to examine whether their assumptions and interpretations among a sample in the US compared with those among a sample of women and men in India. Exposures and risks were identified in the transcripts based on the three structures of the Theory of Gender and Power. Prominent themes that were identified were: (a) sex work initiation, (b) violence between couples, (c) coercive situations, (d) forced sex, (e) married relations, (f) sexual communications, (g) sexual negotiations, (h) alcohol use, (i) post-drinking sex, (j) condom use, (k) client violence, (l) social norms, and (m) marital norms.

RESULTS

Sexual Division of Labor

According to Wingood and DiClemente's (2000) model, in the structure of sexual division of labor, higher poverty levels are one of the main economic exposures that increase both women's vulnerability to HIV and varying levels of violence. From the narratives of women in our study, factors such as lack of education and appropriate vocational skills, combined with the stress of economic constraints, seemed to be the underlying mechanism related to women entering sex work as the sole means of ensuring survival for themselves and their families. One of the respondents described the role of a female relative during a time of severe economic hardship in initiating her into the sex trade:

> In the beginning I had a lot of problems...I did not have money to buy milk for my children. My in-laws were torturing me, there was nobody to take care ....My husband did not take care of me...no parents to turn to..... my "periamma" (mother's sister) took me to Ice House (a place in Chennai)...I waited for a whole day without any food or drink... one man came, fed me, consoled me...He took me to a lodge and had sex with me....and gave me money.... He said he will take care of me and the children. And when he knew that I wanted more money to support my children he introduced me to his friends...and then I started going to them too....

> (Married female, aged 45, illiterate, mother of two, sex worker)

It was also evident that in the 'high demand/low control' sex work environment, brokers and pimps played a vital role in negotiations with male clients that determined women's incomes: "I have not solicited any man directly. All these are handled by the many brokers....clients approach brokers who approach us.... the rate varies... 10% of my earnings go to my broker...." (Married female, aged 35, illiterate, mother of four, sex worker).

In addition, criminalization of sex work in India and fear of violence from police poses further obstacles in women's abilities to control their work environment. As one sex worker described:

> ...if there is a police raid and if we are caught, the client will say that I am his wife. But I generally tell the police the truth fearing physical violence and so they will collect Rs.200 as bribe from me and another Rs.200 from the client too....

> (Married female, aged 35, illiterate, mother of four, sex worker)

However, our data also provide evidence of well-established mutual support systems among sex workers to deal with potentially violent clients, which points to women's efforts to ensure safety in the often dangerous, clandestine sex work environment:

> When the argument continues, they (friends) will knock the door from outside, ask what is happening, and enquire whether it is over. . . . I will tell that man–look they are calling. . . . I will push him and tell him that it is getting late and I am leaving . . . he will say, 'You are trying to run after taking money'. . . . I will say, 'I cannot do anything more, do it yourself'. . . . I close the door and leave the room.

(Widowed female, aged 40, illiterate, no children, sex worker)

While sex workers in Chennai face significant hurdles in their attempts to control their work lives and remain safe, there is evidence of success by some. A few of the sex workers in our study described very firm, scripted sexual negotiation patterns that were executed in advance, while others narrated experiences of being firm with clients during sexual acts. As one women described: "I myself will make them wear Nirodh (a popular brand of condom). I won't accept such people. I will ask them to move or I will move from that place . . . . I have fear as I have to protect my body. . . ." (Widowed female, aged 40, illiterate, no children, sex Worker). There was also evidence of use of covert mechanisms that women used to resist engaging in unwanted sexual practices.

> I don't like to be kissed . . . and will not kiss. So they will harass me by sucking this side and that side and also my neck area . . . I eat "Pan Parag" (brand name of a chewing tobacco) . . . they will ask, 'Is my mouth smelling?' I will say 'Your mouth is not smelling, mine will smell since I am taking "Pan Parag'. . . this way, I will not kiss . . . .

(Married female, aged 35, primary education, no children, sex worker)

Some of the male clients attest to acquiescence to sex workers' demands for condom use: "When I go, they will ask me to wear. Since they are saying, I wear. If I don't listen to them, they won't oblige, so I will wear." (Unmarried male client of sex worker, aged 29, completed primary education). Nevertheless, for many sex workers, violence from

Backs Against the Wall

clients was a significant barrier that created fear and impeded condom negotiation:

> Sometimes when a client physically hurts me, I even cry thinking of what is happening to my life. They will be aggressive and then would ask me to be totally naked, would want to have anal sex–"thirumbi paddu" or they would want me to indulge in activities they have seen in some sex movie. Sometimes they will want me to suck their semen–"vaayila vindhu idhu pannanum" . . . if you see here, a customer has burnt me with a cigarette (she shows her hand) and I have suffered enough . . . .

(Married and deserted, aged 35, illiterate, mother of three, sex worker)

Sexual Division of Power

In Wingood and DiClemente's (2000) model, the structure of sexual division of power focuses on physical exposures such as intimate partner violence and partners with high risk behaviors in addition to other risk factors including use of alcohol, women's perceived lack of control in intimate relationships, and low assertive skills to negotiate condom use that may increase women's vulnerability to HIV. Our findings include the experiences of sex workers as well as other women and men from the community. One respondent expressed her frustration when dealing with violent consequences as a result of condom negotiation with her husband:

> . . . they (the doctors) spoke about "Nirodh"–condom. I used to ask him to bring condom. . . . he used to say that he is clean and that nothing is wrong with him . . . that I am unnecessarily trusting the doctors. He will not bring the condom and when I insisted, he used to abuse me verbally and hit me.

(Married female, aged 28, illiterate, mother of four)

Alcohol use is also an important behavioral risk factor that poses obstacles to safe sexual practices, and we found that this was true for both sex workers and women from the community. While many sex workers admitted using alcohol to overcome inhibition and dull the pain of engaging in sex work, their ability to engage in safe sex and protect themselves was often compromised as a result:

> Someone while having sex with me will remove the Nirodh and do as it is. . . . I would have been drunk and I may not know. Afterwards when I notice and ask him, he will say that he is not able to do it with the Nirodh on, they will force me and have unprotected sex. . . .

(Married female, illiterate, aged 30, mother of three, sex worker)

Narrations from married women also mentioned obstacles to resist unwanted sex that stemmed from alcohol use of their male partners, especially physical violence and accusations of infidelity: "When he is drunk . . . he will accuse me saying, 'you are having a relationship with someone, that is the reason you are not cooperating with me.' Then he will beat me. . . ." (Married female, illiterate, aged 31, mother of one).

Men's narratives also highlighted women's inability to negotiate sex in the context of their own alcohol use and women's fear of physical violence: "She (wife) will not refuse. My wife will give me good company even when I am drunk. She will think since I beat her, she should not refuse. . . . " (Married male, completed primary education, aged 36, wine shop customer, father of five).

One female respondent in our study described her unsuccessful experience in negotiation with her partner who disapproved of practicing safe sex:

> Since he has been traveling, in case he had been to some women, and he is affected, I will be scared of what could happen. So I will tell him to wear one (condom) and he will retort saying that he would slipper me if I suspect him of cheating on me. I am not using any protection with a belief that my husband will not involve in any sexual contact with anyone else. The rest I leave it to God- 'ellam kadavul siddham.'

(Married female, aged 27, completed primary education, no children)

Another respondent in our study reported feeling helpless when trying to negotiate with her husband. He had not only had a second wife, but also visited sex workers frequently. Although fully aware of her own vulnerability and that of his second wife, this woman was unable to assert herself and affect any behavior change in her husband:

He will immediately start a fight and then he will accuse us, saying that we are the ones who are going and sleeping with other men that we are asking about condom use. Because in our community the practice is that women cannot use or bring up the topic of condom use...it is only men who do that. So if we are taught then we ask our husbands to use, then they will be suspicious about us and the fight begins. Then he beats us. . . .

(Married female, aged 31, mother of two)

However, it is important to note that not all women were unsuccessful in their attempts to negotiate sex with their male partners. While power is a critical element in sexual negotiations, there was often a wide range in outcomes depending on the heterogeneity of sexual encounters and the couples' unique sexual behaviors. By both female and male reports of sexual behaviors and practices, it was evident that some women were able to thwart unwanted sex while others were able to refuse sex due to 'legitimate' causes; for example, "If he asks me...when our children are around we could not have sex as there was just one room and so if I was not interested he would also not force me. . . . " (Married female, aged 39, completed primary education, mother of two); and

I will tell that I cannot tolerate the stink and I will refuse. I will tell him that we will have some other day and I will adjust. . . I will tell that I am not feeling well and let's not have today and we will have some other day . . .he will ask why I am not coming along. I will say that I am not well. . . .

(Married female, aged 45, illiterate, mother of four)

Some men also acknowledged certain boundaries of sexual behaviors they would not trespass with their wives: The truth is my wife will not let me have sex with her once I am drunk–naan kudichenna en veetula sekkaadhu. She will be scolding me and in fact, I have to sleep in the platform. (Married male, aged 46, completed primary education, father of four).

One sex worker reported the use of covert and cautious mechanisms when dealing with potentially problematic clients:

If the customers buy and give, I will drink. I will not drink myself.
. . I will see his face, if he is not good I will not drink even that . . . I
will pour it in the bathroom and tell them that I drank it.

(Married female, aged 29, completed primary education, mother of
two, sex worker)

Contrary to other instances where women's alcohol use diminished
women's abilities to negotiate sex, one of the sex workers described her
own use of violence with a client and the use of alcohol as an enabler in
effective initiation and execution of sexual negotiations:

Men would want to have different types of sex–"gents vandhu
pallamurraila irrukannummunu solluvaango." But I do not like all
that. Only when I drink can I fight back and also tell them that I
cannot accept to have sex in the various ways that he has seen in
sex movies. I have in fact hit some people too.

(Married and deserted female, aged 35, illiterate, mother of three, sex
worker)

Cathexis

The structure of cathexis focuses on women's acceptance of traditional social norms, including women's emotional attachments to men
that perpetuate power differentials and deter women from adopting
mechanisms to thwart vulnerability to HIV:

He accepted me as a wife, showered love and affection...I also
started developing "paasam" (affection). . . I will not use condom
with him. He is my husband and I have selected him. Whatever
difficulty or dislike there is, he is after all my husband. . . .

(Married female, aged 41, completed primary education, no children)

Women's implicit acceptance of male violence as normative also
seemed to extend to underplaying the role of physical violence in their
intimate relationships:

We will fight regarding money matters . . . two, three times I have
got beatings from my husband. I would have spoken too much or

quarreled with him. If I ask him anything, he will kick me [but] he won't take cane and beat me. He will kick me at the hip and nothing more than that....

(Married female, aged 35, completed primary education, mother of three)

Women's narratives revealed internalization of traditional norms and almost complete compliance with societal dictates of male normative behavior, including the acceptance of male extra-marital relationships:

Since my husband is a truck driver there will be nirodh (condom) in the truck and he uses it with me ...he always used to say that infections which are spreading will never come to them. 'We (the men) can have "velliya pazhakam" (extramarital relationships) but to prevent any infections, we (men) can use nirodh to prevent them' he tells me whenever he's going to other women. I do not say anything because he has been very open with me and he has not hidden anything from me. There is nothing for me to feel because I know that a man will have these urges when he is going to be away from his wife and it is only natural that he has to go to someone. But the most important thing is that he tells me everything and tells me all the time....

(Married female, aged 22, illiterate, mother of two)

DISCUSSION

This paper has highlighted the many complexities that determine vulnerability to HIV among poor urban women in Chennai, India. The findings from the current study indicate that the Theory of Gender and Power was partially validated in accounting for women's vulnerability to HIV/AIDS in India. In the sexual division of labor construct, lack of economic resources combined with the lack of control in the work environment for sex workers with rampant exploitation from pimps and police seemed to heighten women's vulnerability. This finding was similar to other studies that have underscored the roles played by poverty and police atrocities in sex workers' abilities to control their work lives (Blanchard et al., 2005; Jayasree, 2004; Otutubikey Izugbara, 2005; Pauw & Brener, 2003; Wojcicki & Malala, 2001). However, findings also revealed that strong social and mutually supportive networks and the use of unique covert strategies were vital tools that female sex workers used to protect themselves from the dangers and disadvantages of their occupation, thereby possibly reducing their vulnerability. This finding was also similar to those found in earlier studies (Campbell, 2000; Otutubikey Izugbara; Wojcicki & Malala).

Using the sexual division of power construct, we posited that exposures to partner violence paired with behavioral risk factors such as alcohol use, as well as the lack of perceived control over condom use, would increase women's vulnerability to infection; this was partially supported by the current study. Similar to earlier findings (Asthana & Oostvogels, 1996; Blanchard et al., 2005; Elmore-Meegan, Conroy, & Bernard Agala, 2004; Farley, Baral, Kiremire, & Sezgin, 1998, Miller, 2002; Otutubikey Izugbara, 2005; Wojcicki & Malala, 2001), intimate partner violence and client violence in the case of sex workers were important factors that limited women's abilities to engage in safe sex behaviors. Further, lack of control in relationships with aggressive clients and in the face of accusations of infidelity by suspicious spouses were important determinants that impinged on women's abilities to protect themselves. However, even under these adverse circumstances, there was clear evidence of some women's ability to engage in effective sexual negotiations, decline unwanted sexual contact, insist on condom use, and adopt safer behaviors as in some earlier studies. Asthana and Oostvogels also observed that although the risks for sex workers in Chennai are high for violence, these women are sometimes better able to assert and protect themselves than married women given their strong informal support networks. George's (1998) study reported similar findings from Mumbai, India, where women negotiated the nature of sexual outcomes under specific circumstances, instead of outright refusals which had the risk of resulting in violence and/or forced sex. Interestingly, similar to findings from other studies among sex workers that found evidence of male acquiescence to female controlled sexual negotiation (Campbell, 2000; Cusik, 1998; Sanders, 2004), some male clients in our study also seemed to accept sex workers' terms of sexual negotiation.

Within the structure of cathexis construct, it was expected that higher levels of acceptability of traditional norms would indicate lowered abilities to engage in sexual negotiation and increased vulnerability to HIV/AIDS; this was completely supported by the findings of the current study.

Findings from application of the Theory of Gender and Power to examine women's vulnerability to HIV/AIDS in India revealed that vulnerability was not universal and, despite formidable obstacles, many women displayed ingenuity in exercising personal agency and power in their abilities to negotiate safe sex practices. Despite adverse circumstances, many women in our study seemed to display strength when engaging in a wide range of behaviors that symbolized resistance to male power, whether by use of covert or overt strategies to safeguard their health and resist violence.

This study draws on contributions to the existing literature by using a theoretical model to examine the various factors that are associated with women's increased vulnerability to violence and HIV/AIDS. Women's narratives help provide a richer and deeper understanding of the linkages between partner violence, the dynamics of sexual negotiations between females and males, and vulnerability to HIV. However, caution needs to be exercised when generalizing findings from this study, especially in light of our small sample size and non-random sampling methodology. Also, because this study focused on socio-economically disadvantaged populations, the findings cannot be generalized to other populations in Chennai or elsewhere in India. Replicating this study using this theoretical framework in other sites in India may provide additional insights into culture-specific factors that could be indicative of possibly reducing women's vulnerability to HIV/AIDS.

SUMMARY

Sexual encounters between women and men hinge on unequal power relations between the genders (Taylor, 1995). Complexities of the sexual negotiation between married couples also involve familial and economic situations based on cultural norms and the resources available to them individually and jointly, in addition to differential sexual norms and expectations (George, 1998). While economic hardships, power differentials, victimization, and societal norms play a major role in limiting options for women to assert their sexual rights, it is amply clear that it may be dangerous to assume unitary responses in all heterosexually-related sexual encounters. Our study clearly underscores the need to recognize women's agency in resisting violence and/or forced sex from men, either sexual clients or husbands, as well as women's attempts to safeguard their own health.

The findings from this study have several implications for intervention. Targeting boys and men in discourses of sexual equality, power and control, and safe sex are important steps in ensuring reduced vulnerability of women to violence and disease. In short, men need to change. Empowerment also needs to be viewed as a broader societal process that addresses gender imbalances in all spheres, especially the economic arena. Importantly, empowerment of women to gain control of their sexual lives will necessitate a radical departure in the manner in which gender relations are constructed, elimination of economic dependency on men, and rethinking discriminatory cultural norms through advocacy and education (Heise & Elias, 1995). This is particularly relevant for sex workers and wives involved in abusive relationships whose personal safety may be compromised if they engage in sexual negotiations with their partners. Hence, AIDS prevention programs also need to take into account the complex dynamics of abusive relationships, and stress training and skill-building for women who wish to lead violence-free lives (Davila, 2002; El-Bassel et al., 2000). Finally, if women are to exercise their sexual rights without fear of reprisals from their male partners, it is imperative to place female-controlled preventive methods in women's hands.

REFERENCES

Acevedo, M. J. (2000). Battered immigrant Mexican women's perspectives regarding abuse and help-seeking. *Journal of Multicultural Social Work, 8*, 243-282.

Adkins, L. (1995). *Gendered work.* Philadelphia, PA: Open University Press.

Amaro, H. (1995). Love, sex, and power: Considering women's realities in HIV prevention. *American Pyschologist, 50*, 437-447.

Asthana, S., & Oostvogels, R. (1996). Community participation in HIV prevention: Problems and prospects for community based strategies among female sex workers in Madras. *Social Science Medicine, 43*(2), 133-148.

Bhave, G., Lindan, C. P., Hudes, E. S., Desai, S., Wagle, U., Tripathi, S. P., et al. (1995). Impact of an intervention on HIV, sexually transmitted diseases, and condom use among sex workers in Bombay, India. *AIDS, 9*(Suppl 1), S21-S30.

Blanchard, J. F., O'Neil, J., Ramesh, B. M., Bhattacharjee, P., Orchard, T., & Moses, S. (2005). Understanding the social and cultural contexts of female sex workers in Karnataka, India: Implications for prevention of HIV infection. *Journal of Infectious Diseases, 191*(Suppl 1), 139-146.

Campbell, C. (2000). Selling sex in the time of AIDS: The psycho-social context of condom use by sex workers on a South African mine. *Social Science and Medicine, 50*, 479-494.

Celentano, D., Sivaram, S., Mayer, K., Krishnan, A., Murugavel, K., Go, V., et al. (2001, October). *HIV/STD burden in urban slums of South India.* Paper presented at the 6th International Congress on AIDS in Asia and the Pacific, Melbourne, Australia.

Connell, R. W. (1987). *Gender and power: Society, the person, and sexual politics.* Palo Alto, CA: Stanford University Press.

Cusik, L. (1998). Non-use of condoms by prostitute women. *AIDS Care, 10*(2), 133-146.

Davila, Y. R. (2000). Hispanic women and AIDS: Gendered risk factors and clinical implications. *Issues in Mental Health Nursing, 21,* 635-646.

Davila, Y. R. (2002). Influence of abuse on condom negotiation among Mexican-American women involved in abusive relationships. *Journal of the Association of Nurses in AIDS Care, 13*(6), 46-56.

Dunkle K. L., Jewkes, R. K., Brown, H. C., Gray, G. E., McIntryre, J. A., & Harlow, S. D. (2004). Gender-basedviolence, relationship power, and risk of HIV infection in women attending antenatal clinics in South Africa. *Lancet, 363*(9419), 1415-21.

El-Bassel, N., Gilbert, L., Krishnan, S., Schilling, R., Gaeta, T., Purpura, S., et al. (1998). Partner violence and sexual HIV-risk behaviors among women in an inner-city emergency department. *Violence and Victims, 13*(4), 377-393.

El-Bassel, N., Gilbert, L., Rajah, V., Foleno, A., & Frye, V. (2000). Fear and violence: Raising the HIV stakes. *AIDS Education and Prevention, 12*(2), 154-70.

Elmore-Meegan, M., Conroy, R. M., & Bernard Agala, C. (2004). Sex workers in Kenya, numbers of clients and associated risks: An exploratory survey. *Reproductive Health Matters, 12*(23), 50-57.

Farley, M., Baral, I., Kiremire, M., & Sezgin, U. (1998). Prostitution in five countries: Violence and post-traumatic stress disorder. *Feminism & Psychology, 8*(4), 405-426.

Gangakhedkar, R. R., Bentley, M. E., Divekar, A. D., Gadkari, D., Mehendale, S. M., Shepherd,M. E., et al. (1997). Spread of HIV infection in married monogamous women in India. *Journal of the American Medical Association, 278,* 2090-2092.

George, A. (1998). Differential perspectives of men and women in Mumbai, India on sexual relations and negotiations within marriage. *Reproductive Health Matters, 6*(12), 87-96.

Go, V. F., Sethulakshmi, C. J., Bentley, M. E., Sivaram, S., Srikrishnan, A. K., Solomon, S., et al. (2003). When HIV-prevention messages and gender norms clash: The impact of domestic violence on women's HIV risk in slums of Chennai, India. *AIDS and Behavior, 7*(3), 263-272.

Gupta, G. R., Weiss, E., & Whelan, D. (1995). Male-female inequalities result in submission to high-risk sex in many societies. Special report: women and HIV. *AIDS Analysis Africa, 5*(4), 8-9.

Hassouneh-Phillips, D. (2001). American Muslim women's experiences of leaving abusive relationships. *Health Care for Women International, 22,* 415-432.

Heise, L. L. (1993). Reproductive freedom and violence against women: Where are the intersections? *The Journal of Law, Medicine, and Ethics, 21*(3), 206-216.

Heise, L. L., & Elias, C. (1995). Transforming aids prevention to meet women's needs: A focus on developing countries. *Social Science and Medicine, 40,* 931-943.

Holland, J., & Ramazanoglu, C. (1992). Risk, power, and the possibility of pleasure: Young women and safer sex. *AIDS Care, 4*(3), 273-283.

Jayasree, A. K. (2004). Searching for justice for body and self in a coercive environment: Sex work in Kerala, India. *Reproductive Health Matters, 12*(23), 58-67.

Jinich, S., Paul, J., & Stall, R. (1998). Childhood sexual abuse and HIV-risk taking behavior among gay and bisexual men. *AIDS and Behavior, 2*(1), 41-51.

Koenig, M. A., Lutalo, T., Zhao, F., Nalugoda, F., Kiwanuka, N, Wabwire-Mangen, F., et al. (2004). Coercive sex in rural Uganda: Prevalence and associated risk factors. *Social Science and Medicine, 58*(4), 787-98.

Koenig, M. A., Lutalo, T., Zhao, F., Nalugoda, F., Wabwire-Mangen, F., Kiwanuka, N., et al. (2003). Domestic violence in rural Uganda: Evidence from a community-based study. *Bulletin of the World Health Organization, 81*(1), 53-60.

Lodico, M., & DiClemente, R. J. (1994). The association between childhood sexual abuse and prevalence of HIV-related risk behaviors. *Clinical Pediatrics, 8*, 498-502.

Majumdar, B. (2004). An exploration of socioeconomic, spiritual, and family support among HIV-positive women in India. *The Journal of the Association of Nurses in AIDS Care, 15*(3), 37-46.

Maman, S., Campbell, J., Sweat, M. D., & Gielen, A. C. (2000). The intersections of HIV and violence: Directions for future research and interventions. *Social Science and Medicine, 50*, 459-478.

Martin, S. L., & Curtis, S. (2004). Commentary: Gender-based violence and HIV/AIDS: Recognising links and acting on evidence. *The Lancet, 363*(9419), 1410-1411.

Martin, S. L., Kilgallen, B., Tsui, A. O., Maitra, K., Singh, K. K., & Kupper, L. L. (1999). Sexual behaviors and reproductive health outcomes: associations with wife abuse in India. *The Journal of the American Medical Association, 282*, 1967-1972.

McDonnell, K. A., Gielen, A. C., & O'Campo, P. (2003). Does HIV status make a difference in the experience of lifetime abuse? Descriptions of lifetime abuse and its context among low-income urban women. *Journal of Urban Health, 80*(3), 494-509.

Miller, J. (2002). Violence and coercion in Sri Lanka's commercial sex industry: Intersections of gender, sexuality, culture, and the law. *Violence Against Women, 8*(9), 1044-1073.

Monahan, J. L., Miller, L. C., & Rothspan, S. (1997). Power and intimacy: on the dynamics of risky sex. *Health Communication, 9*, 303-321.

Muhr, T. (1997). *Atlas TI 4.1.* Berlin: Scientific Software Development.

National AIDS Control Organization. (2004). *HIV estimates- 2004.* Retrieved June 1, 2006 from, http://www.nacoonline.org/facts_hivestimates04.htm.

Newmann, S., Sarin, P., Kumarasamy, N., Amalraj, E., Rogers, M., Madhivanan, P., et al. (2000). Marriage, monogamy and HIV: a profile of HIV-infected women in south India. *International Journal of STD and AIDS, 11*, 250-253.

Otutubikey Izugbara, C. (2005). "Ashawo suppose shine her eyes": Female sex workers and sex work risks in Nigeria. *Health, Risk & Society, 7*(2), 141-159.

Pauw, I., & Brener, L. (2003). "You are just whores - you can't be raped": Barriers to safer sex practices among women street sex workers in Cape Town. *Culture, Health & Sexuality, 5*(6), 465-481.

Pulerwitz, J., Amaro, H., De Jong, W., & Gortmaker, S. L. (2002). Relationship power, condom use and HIV risk among women in the USA. *AIDS Care, 14*(6), 789-800.

Raj, A., Silverman, J. G., Wingood, G. M., & DiClemente, R. J. (1999). Prevalence and correlates of relationship abuse among a community sample of low-income African-American women. *Violence Against Women, 5*(3), 272-291.

Rao Gupta, G. (2002). How men's power over women fuels the HIV epidemic. *British Medical Journal, 324*(7331), 183-184.

Rao Gupta, G., & Weiss, E. (1993). *Women and AIDS: Developing a new health strategy.* ICRW Policy Series. Washington, DC: International Center for Research on Women.

Ravindran, S. T. K., & Balasubramanian, P. (2004). "Yes" to abortion but "No" to sexual rights: The paradoxical reality of married women in rural Tamil Nadu, India. *Reproductive Health Matters, 12*(23), 88-99.

Rose, L. E., Campbell, J. C., & Kub, J. (2000). The role of social support and family relationships in women's responses to battering. *Health Care for Women International, 21*, 27-39.

Sanders, T. (2004). A continuum of risk? The management of health, physical, and emotional risks by female sex workers. *Sociology of Health and Illness, 26*(5), 557-574.

Santow, G. (1995). Social roles and physical health: the case of female disadvantage in poor countries. *Social Science Medicine, 40*(2), 147-161.

Shrotri A, Shankar A. V., Sutar, S., Joshi, A., Suryawanshi, N., Pisal, H., et al. (2003). Awareness of HIV/AIDS and household environment of pregnant women in Pune, India. *International Journal of STD and AIDS, 14*(12), 835-839.

Taylor, B. M. (1995). Gender-power relations and safe sex negotiation. *Journal of Advanced Nursing, 22*, 687-693.

Venkataramana, C. B. S., & Sarada, P. V. (2001). Extent and speed of spread of HIV infection in India through the commercial sex networks: a perspective. *Tropical Medicine and International Health, 6*(12), 1040-1061.

Wingood, G. M., & DiClemente, R. J. (1997). The effects of an abusive primary partner on the condom use and sexual negotiation practices of African-American women. *American Journal of Public Health, 87*, 1016-1018.

Wingood, G. M., & DiClemente, R. J. (1998). Rape among African American women: sexual, psychological, and social correlates predisposing survivors to risk of STD/HIV. *Journal of Women's Health, 7*, 77-84.

Wingood, G. M., & DiClemente, R. J. (1998). Partner influences and gender-related factors associated with noncondom use among young adult African-American women. *American Journal of Community Psychology, 26*, 29-51.

Wingood, G. M., & DiClemente, R. J. (2000). Application of the Theory of Gender and Power to examine HIV-related exposures, risk factors, and effective interventions for women. *Health Education and Behavior, 27*(5), 539-565.

UNAIDS. (2004). *Women and AIDS fact sheet: UNAIDS epidemic update.* Retrieved December 1, 2004 from, http://womenandaids.unaids.org

Wojcicki, J. M., & Malala, J. (2001). Condom use, power and HIV/AIDS risk: Sex-workers bargain for survival in Hillbrow/Joubert Park/Berea, Johannesburg. *Social Science & Medicine, 53*(1), 99-121.

World Health Organization. (2000). *Women of south-east Asia. A health profile.* Retrieved November 24, 2004 from, http://w3.whosea.org/women/bookreleasef.htm

ACKNOWLEDGMENTS

Funding support: National Institute for Mental Health Grant U10 681543-01 & Fogarty International Center: Grant # 2 D 4 3 TW000010-17-AITRP. The authors would also like to thank Kathy McCloskey, Suzanne Maman, and Muzamillah Jeelani for their helpful comments on earlier versions of this paper.

NOTES

1. Before interviews were conducted, participants were informed that referrals were available, informed about the inherent psychological and social risks to data provision, and asked for both verbal and written consent. Battering and other forms of widespread violence against women are common in India, and given the existing social networks in the slums where participants lived and the geographical proximity of residential units, it seemed difficult to keep instances of battering private. As such we found that information provided by participants was not new or revelatory in any way, nor did revealing this information to interviewers seem to increase the risk of future battering incidents. The overarching study is in its 6th year and we have had no adverse events reported as a result of women's disclosures concerning the violence in their lives.

Submitted: May 3, 2005
Revised: January 19, 2007
Revised: May 8, 2007
Accepted: May 26, 2007

The Ecology of Intimate Partner Violence: Theorized Impacts on Women's Use of Violence

Marilyn Sitaker

Intimate partner violence (IPV) has been described as the physical and verbal expression of a dominant person's attempt to exert control over an intimate partner (a current or former spouse, boyfriend or girlfriend, same-sex partner, or date; Bachman, 2000; DeKeseredy, 2000; Gordon, 2000). IPV may include physical beatings, verbal abuse, emotional or psychological abuse, withholding financial support, sexual abuse, imposing social isolation, or neglecting to provide a dependent spouse with necessary food, safe shelter, and clothing. While men can be victims of IPV, overwhelming evidence suggests that women are at much higher risk than men for IPV, and are more likely than men to suffer IPV-related injuries (Malloy, McCloskey, Grigsby, & Gardner, 2003; Tjaden & Thoennes, 1998, 2000a, 2000b).

IPV has emerged as an important public health issue due to its health consequences. These include IPV-related injuries, abuse during pregnancy, IPV-related homicides and suicides, and chronic mental health conditions such as depression, anxiety, and post-traumatic stress disorder (Campbell et al., 2002). Beyond associated health care costs and lost productivity due to mental and physical disability, IPV exacts a toll on society by increasing a dependent child's likelihood of becoming an adult victim or a perpetrator of IPV, thus perpetuating the problem across generations (Guille, 2004; Simons & Johnson, 1998).

The controversy over the reasons behind recent increases in women's arrest for domestic violence is a result of competing hypotheses, yet no known research has definitively shown that the increase in women's arrests is anything but a poor implementation of recent public policy changes, most notably the advent of mandatory/preferred arrest laws. As a strategic framework for the amelioration of IPV, the public health problem-solving model offers a unique perspective: an emphasis on prevention and a focus on populations as opposed to individuals. This approach begins with a definition of the nature and scope of the problem. The next step involves a search for underlying causes and the mechanisms by which they operate. In the public health model, the search for underlying causes goes beyond the role of biological and psychological factors to include geographic, environmental, and social influences. An understanding of both risk and protective factors is sought, with priority given to those causal factors that are modifiable. However, variations in risk by non-modifiable factors such as age, gender, and race/ethnicity are important to quantify because they can help identify sub-groups at higher risk (Campbell, 2000; Saltzman, 2000). Finally, the findings from etiologic studies are used to develop interventions, which are then evaluated for their effectiveness. Wolfe and Jaffe (1999) describe public health interventions as those that act "along a continuum of possible harm: (1) primary prevention to reduce the incidence of the problem before it occurs, (2) secondary prevention to decrease the prevalence after early signs of the problem, and (3) tertiary prevention to intervene once the problem is already clearly evident and causing harm" (p. 133). The issue of women's use of violence within intimate relationships is thus embedded in global population findings that show women, compared to men, constitute but a small subset of perpetrators. The aim of this paper is to describe the etiology of IPV, using the social-ecological framework developed by Heise (1998) to categorize research findings from multiple disciplines according to the level of social organization at which they operate. Next, evidence-based strategies will be reviewed according to the sphere of influence in the social ecological model, and their place on the prevention continuum. In this paper, primary prevention refers to efforts that prevent victimization and perpetration of IPV before it occurs, and secondary prevention refers to interventions that interrupt the cycle of IPV and prevent its re-occurrence. Finally, the relevance within each level of the model to women's use of violence will be discussed.

ETIOLOGY OF IPV

Over the past 20 years, theories regarding the underlying causes of IPV have been shaped by research conducted within the disciplines of psychology, sociology, and criminology. Academic theorists tended to emphasize individual explanations for IPV (e.g., men beat women because of psychopathology or poor impulse control) while feminist activists emphasized social/political explanations (e.g., battering results from historical construction of the patriarchal family and gender-power inequalities). Academic researchers' failure to account for gendered differences in social power resulted in theories that could not explain why women were disproportionately the target of male violence, and allowed the mistaken assumption that women are violent like men to flourish. Yet by emphasizing patriarchy as a causal mechanism (to the exclusion of individual factors), feminist theory failed to explain why not all men who grow up with social affirmation of male entitlement become perpetrators of IPV (Heise, 1998), or why a small subset of women are indeed primary IPV perpetrators. The biases specific to a variety of academic disciplines combined with the ideological stance of feminist activists precluded the development of an integrated theory on which intervention programs could be based.

Developing an Ecologic Framework for Understanding IPV

A seminal paper written in 1998 by Heise sought to reconcile the individual-factor perspective with the social-cultural perspective, using an ecological framework to integrate the array of personal, situational, and social factors that interact to predict IPV. While Heise was not the first to use ecological theory to describe interpersonal violence (e.g., Grigsby & Hartman, 1997), her work was groundbreaking in that it sought to organize existing research on predictive factors according to their level of influence in the social ecological model. Heise incorporated findings from research on many types of interpersonal violence, including international and cross-cultural studies. By broadening her scope, she was able to find underlying factors operating at outer layers of the social ecological model that have not traditionally been studied by North American IPV researchers.

The social ecological model used by Heise (1998) is drawn as four concentric circles (see Figure 1) that show each level of causality as embedded within higher levels, and to reflect the interaction between factors at various levels. The innermost circle represents biological, demographic, and personal history factors that each individual (victim or perpetrator, male or female) brings to his or her behavior in relationships. The next layer focuses on interpersonal relationships, the immediate context in which abuse takes place and the influence of relationships with family and friends. The third layer represents the institutions and social structures in the community: the neighborhood, workplace, justice system, social networks, and peer groups in which the relationship is embedded. The fourth, outermost circle is the economic and social environment, representing the general views and attitudes that permeate the culture at large. Heise discussed ways in which the ecological framework could be applied to the study of individual factors associated with IPV, or applied to cross-cultural studies to better elucidate the expression of multilevel factors across various settings.

It was not until 2002 that an attempt was made to further investigate factors at all levels of the social ecological model (Jewkes, 2002). Like Heise (1998), Jewkes notes that our understanding of the social context in which IPV occurs has been limited by past research confined largely to North American studies that use samples drawn from batterer's treatment or women's shelters. Over the past decade, however, well-designed studies that focus on both women and men have been conducted in developing countries, greatly expanding the research base. Koenig, Ahmed, Hossain, and Mozumder (2003) further underscored Jewkes' analysis of the current state of knowledge in an extensive literature review that accompanied their study of women's status and domestic violence in rural Bangladesh.

The following section reviews factors discussed by Heise (1998), Jewkes (2002), and Koenig et al. (2003) at each of level of the social ecological model that increase the likelihood of IPV. Few studies investigated the factors that increase the likelihood that a woman will abuse her partner, whether as a primary perpetrator or in response to her own abuse, mostly due to the low base-rates of female perpetrators within the populations of interest. Thus, most research is directed toward male perpetrators, and rightly so. Where applicable, possible application to women's use of violence will be noted.

INDIVIDUAL: PERSONAL HISTORY

Demographic Factors

As noted above, sociological studies have found gender to be the strongest demographic predictor of IPV; males have higher perpetration rates for interpersonal violence of all types, including sexual assault and IPV as well as higher rates of criminality in general. Rates of violence also vary by age, with higher rates reported among young adults (Hastings & Hamberger, 1997). People of color and/or minority ethnicity also report higher rates of victimization (Gelles, 1993; Smith, 1990;

FIGURE 1. Levels of Influence in the Socio-Ecological Model (adapted from Heise, 1998).

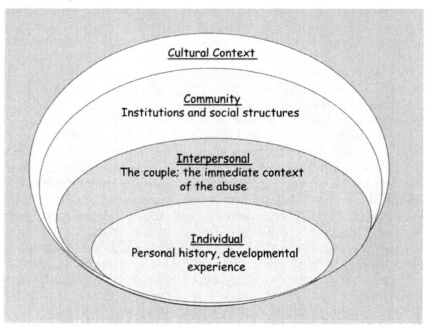

Straus, Gelles, & Steinmetz, 1980; Tjaden & Thoennes 2000a, 2000b). As with many disparities in adverse health-related outcomes, some of the differences in IPV by race and ethnicity can be explained by socioeconomic status (SES; Hastings & Hamberger, 1997). Gelles suggested that the increased stress and social isolation experienced by those of lower SES lead to higher rates of violence, although study limitations have made it hard to tell whether stress and isolation are a cause or a result of violence. While IPV occurs within every SES strata, cross-cultural studies from the U.S., India, and Nicaragua (Bachman & Saltzman, 1995; Ellsberg, Pena, Herrera, Liljestrand, & Winkvist, 1999; Gelles & Straus, 1998; Hotaling & Sugarman, 1986, 1990; Martin, Tsui, Maitra, & Marinshaw, 1999; Ratner, 1993; Rodriguez, Lasch, Chandra, & Lee, 2001; Vest, Catlin, Chen, & Brownson, 2003) show an increased risk of frequent and severe violence associated with poverty.

Abuse in Childhood

As mentioned above, experiencing or witnessing abuse as a child has been widely demonstrated to increase the likelihood of violence in adulthood. Sons of battered women are more likely to become IPV perpetrators (Abrahams, Jewkes, & Laubscher, 1999; Ellsberg et al., 1999), daughters are more likely to become victims (Abrahams et al.; Hotaling & Sugarman, 1986, 1990; Jewkes, Penn-Kekana, & Levin, 2002), and children of both genders are more likely to be involved in the criminal justice system (Hotaling & Sugarman, 1986, 1990). This relationship has been demonstrated in studies from the U.S. (Caesar, 1988; Hotaling & Sugarman, 1986; Kalmuss, 1984; Straus & Gelles, 1990) and other developing countries (Ellsberg et al.; Jewkes et al.; Martin et al., 1999). While the mechanism by which childhood victimization translates into IPV in adulthood is unclear (Hotaling & Sugarman, 1986, 1990), one might speculate that experiencing abuse in the home teaches children that it is normal to use violence to establish power in relationships, as well as communicates social norms about the appropriateness of using violence toward family members and others.

Heavy Substance Use

Heavy alcohol use increases the risk of violence in general, including IPV (Cruz & Peralta, 2001; Kyriacou, McCabe, Anglin, Lapesarde, & Winer, 1998; McCauley et al., 1995), although not all studies demonstrate these findings (Hoffman, Demo, & Edwards, 1994). Alcohol's role in IPV has been explained as a loss of inhibitions and impaired ability to respond to social cues (Caetano, Schafer, & Cunradi, 2001). However, anthropological studies suggest that the relationship between violence and alcohol use is dependent upon cultural context. Gelles (1974) suggested that drunkenness serves as a "time out" from social norms, during which IPV perpetrators, especially men, may use violence because they are not held responsible for their behavior, either by themselves or others (Testa & Leonard, 2001). A number of cross cultural studies have found both drugs and alcohol to be associated with increased risk of physical and sexual IPV for both perpetrators and victims (Jewkes et al., 2002; Koenig et al., 2003; Rao, 1997; van der Straten et al., 1998; Watts, Keough, Ndlovu, & Kwaramba, 1998).

Status and Autonomy of Women

A number of researchers have studied the empowerment of women as a protective factor against IPV (El-Zantaty, Hussein, Shawky, Way, & Kishor, 1996 Jejeebhoy & Cook, 1997; Profamilia, 1995; Schuler, Hashimi, Riley, & Akhter, 1996). Higher levels of education have been associated with decreased risk of female victimization, where "education confers social empowerment via social networks, self-confidence, and an ability to use information and resources in society" (Jewkes et al., 2002, p. 1425). The relationship between IPV and women's education is not straightforward, however. In South African and North American studies, only women at the lowest and highest levels of education were protected from violence (Department of Health, 2003; Straus et al., 1980). Apparently, it is not until a certain educational threshold is reached, either low or high, that the effect of education influences IPV risk.

INTERPERSONAL:
COUPLES, FAMILIES, AND NEIGHBORS

Marital Conflict

Discord among intimate partners is a strong predictor of abuse (Hotaling & Sugarman, 1990; Hoffman et al., 1994). The frequency of verbal disagreements and high levels of conflict are strongly associated with physical violence (Hoffman et al.; Jewkes et al., 2002; Straus et al., 1980). Risk of IPV is particularly high for female victimization when conflicts occur over finances, challenges to male privilege, perceived transgressions of female gender roles, or a failure to conform to cultural stereotypes of good womanhood (Jewkes et al.). For male perpetrators, transgressions may include not obeying him, talking back, not having dinner ready on time, failing to care for the children or the home according to some standard, going somewhere without permission, refusing sex, or expressing suspicions of infidelity (Heise, 2002). A recent qualitative study by Winstock, Eisikovits, and Gelles (2002) explored the meaning that male perpetrators attach to their use of violence, and found that these men felt they had the right to protect and maintain their relationship as well as their authority, and indeed felt that society expected them to do so. The researchers concluded that these men felt entitled and obligated to use violence to reestablish the balance of power in their favor However, cross-cultural studies make it clear that what is perceived to be a gender role transgression varies by cultural setting. For example, in India disputes over dowry, female sterility, and not producing a male child increase the risk of male IPV perpetration (Rao, 1997), while in South Africa women drinking alcohol, having other sexual partners, or criticizing their partner's drinking were associated with increased risk (Jewkes et al.). Data from Coleman and Straus (1986) point to the dynamic of marital conflict in the presence of asymmetrical power structure: conflicts that occur in more egalitarian relationships are less likely to escalate into physical violence.

Decision-Making and Control of Resources in the Family

Patterns of household decision-making reflect the interpersonal dynamics between men and women in heterosexual relationships. Coleman and Strauss (1986) found that females were victimized in 11% of families in which the male considered himself to be the head of the household with primary decision making authority, compared with 3% of families where partners were more egalitarian. Further, results from an ecologic study involving 30 states found that violence toward women was higher (6.2%) in states where a belief in male authority in family decision-making was strongly endorsed compared to those states with more egalitarian views (3.1%; Straus, 1994).

Cross-cultural studies have also found an increase in IPV when family decision-making is controlled by men (Leung, Leung, Lam & Ho, 1999; Levinson, 1989; Orpinas, 1999). A study in the Philippines found that while lower levels of household wealth and urban residence were moderately associated with IPV, the strongest predictor was household decision-making patterns (Hindin & Adair, 2002). When men dominated major household decisions, women's risk of IPV was 2.7 times greater than women living in households where decision-making was shared equally. However, when women dominated household decisions, their risk of IPV was 3.8 times greater. Overall, 25% of women reported IPV when no household decisions were made jointly, compared to 6% of women living in households making joint decisions (Hindin & Adair).

The association between earning power and IPV is complex and varies by cultural setting. In a South African study, women living in the poorest households were protected from IPV if their main source of income was external to the couple (Jewkes et al., 2002), while a Nicaraguan study (Ellsberg et al., 1999) found that financial independence was not protective for women, unlike findings from studies in Southern India (Schuler et al., 1996) and Bangladesh (Rao, 1997). Indeed, working women in Canada whose partners did not work experienced higher levels of IPV (Jewkes, 2002). These findings suggest that inequality in earning power between male-female couples in the context of poverty may be a stronger predictor of male IPV perpetration than absolute income; however, the relationship of earning power to women's use of violence is largely unknown, at least outside the general context of poverty. In addition, SES needs to be contextualized within the cultural meanings attached to earning power and gender.

The mediation of earning power and gender through the social construction of masculinity was first discussed by Gelles (1974), who postulated that male IPV perpetrators were unable to live up to some criterion of successful manhood through earning power. Bourgois (1996) described adolescent Puerto Rican males in New York City slums who felt caught between the masculine ideal of honor set forth by their families and the consumerism associated with successful manhood in the U.S. With limited opportunities for employment, neither cultural script was attainable and their concept of masculine identity was reshaped to emphasize criminal activity, drug use, and misogynistic attitudes and actions toward women. Thus, some men may experience lack of earning power as a threat to their gender identity and substitute violence toward women as a means to re-establish masculinity (Jewkes et al., 2002; Levinson, 1989).

On the other hand, Levinson's (1989) cross-cultural study found female victimization was more prevalent in societies where men control the family wealth. Male dominance in decision-making (discussed above) and divorce restrictions placed on women were also strongly predictive of IPV. Levinson suggested that the association between men's economic control and female victimization was mediated through the exercise of male authority in the home and societal restrictions on women's access to divorce. A recent study by Jejeebhoy and Cook (1997) found that a wife's control over resources significantly lowered her risk of IPV, although further analysis once again revealed this relationship to be moderated by community norms. A women's autonomy was more strongly protective in the southern Indian state of Tamil Nadu than in the more culturally conservative state of Uttar Pradesh (Jejeebhoy & Cook). Hinden (2000) provides explanations for why earning power may either lower or increase a woman's risk of IPV:

It is theoretically plausible that women's economic empowerment through the process of development may be linked to IPV. On the one hand, women who earn an income and help themselves and their families have means to get out of a bad marriage or not to marry at all. When women have more options, this should decrease the likelihood of their being in an abusive relationship . . . poor women are often most vulnerable to violence because they are most exposed to the risk of violence and least able to remove themselves from violent situations. On the other hand, women's economic empowerment may promote male insecurity and feelings of economic inadequacy, leading to more violence in relationships. (Hinden, 2000, p. 1517)

Status Incompatibility

Theoretical work on the social construction of gender suggests that certain social practices are designed to differentiate men from women; these include gender division of labor inside and outside the household, the tendency for men to marry down and women to marry up, and greater social and economic rewards accorded to men's work (Connell, 1987; South & Spitze, 1994; Williams, 1995). Within U.S. culture, it is considered "normal" for a man to have higher educational and occupational status than his female partner. Status incompatibility refers to couples who deviate from the expected pattern. Hornung, McCullough, and Sugimoto (1981) were among the first to investigate the role of status inconsistency in risk of IPV. Using data from a state-wide telephone survey of married Kentucky women, they compared the occupational level and educational status of the respondent and her male partner with her self-reported perpetration of violence by either partner, and found that couples in which the women was educationally incompatible with her husband, particularly if her attainments were low compared to his, suffered from higher rates of violence, especially life-threatening violence. Conversely, Anderson's (1997) analysis of data from the National Survey of Families and Households found that men in positions of low income status relative to their partners were more likely to perpetrate violence compared to men with earnings on par with their partners. This study also demonstrated an association between elements of the structural environment (age, race, and cohabiting status) and men's perpetration of violence that remained strong after taking status incompatibility into account. In explaining the implication of her findings concerning these interactions, Anderson suggests that the social construction of masculinity requires men to demonstrate their manliness through attainment of educational and occupational prestige. Men who have lower access to symbols of achievement, such as young men and men of color, turn to violence, which is clearly associated with masculinity in the U.S. culture.

Social Support from Family and Friends

As with many health issues, social support appears to be a protective factor against IPV in several cross cultural studies (Counts, Brown, & Campbell, 1992; International Clinical Epidemiologist's Network, 2000). Rao (1997) found that the presence of a wife's brothers was inversely related to reported IPV in South India. Similarly, a study in Cambodia found that the rate of reported violence was 50% lower for couples who resided with the wife's parents, compared to those who did not (Nelson & Zimmerman, 1996). In a comparative study of IPV in 16 non-European cultures, Counts et al. (1992) concluded that family and friends may lessen the risk of IPV by enhancing a woman's self-esteem, making her feel valued, serving as a sounding board for domestic problems, or offering practical assistance. Further, the strongest predictor of societies with low levels of IPV is whether social norms mandate family and friends to intervene if a woman is harassed or beaten. Conversely, social isolation, indicated by infrequent interaction with friends and relatives as well as a lack of participation in public events, has been shown in a number of studies to be both a precursor and a result of abuse (Dobash & Dobash, 1979; Gelles, 1974). Abusive men tend to restrict women's movements and limit their contact with others outside the home. This isolation results in a gradual withdrawal from family and friends on the woman's part, and in "compassion fatigue" on the part of family and friends (Heise, 1998).

COMMUNITY:
INSTITUTIONS AND SOCIAL STRUCTURES

Unemployment/Low Income

O'Campo et al. (1995) were among the first to examine the effects of community-level factors on IPV. They re-analyzed data from a Baltimore (MD) study of physical violence toward pregnant women perpetrated by a male partner, and found that neighborhood characteristics, such as median income level, unemployment rate, and ratio of renters to homeowners, were predictive of IPV. The findings suggest that living in a neighborhood with high unemployment rates and low average income levels may increase risk of IPV apart from risks associated with personal levels of income. The findings of this study were replicated by Cunradi, Caetano, Clark, and Shafer (2000), where it was found that black couples living in impoverished neighborhoods were at higher risk of male-to-female partner violence, and female-to-male partner violence was higher for both black and white couples living in impoverished neighborhoods.

Status of Women

Levinson's (1989) analysis of aggregated data on small scale societies found that societal indicators of female autonomy, such as lack of divorce restrictions, more egalitarian household relationships, and female work groups, were important in protecting women from abuse by husbands. Counts et al. (1992) presented evidence from 16 non-European cultures demonstrating that community-level sanctions against severe wife beating were an important factor in keeping levels of wife beating contained. Finally, the Activa project showed that women who have authority and power outside the family experience lower likelihood of violence at the hands of their male partners (Orpinas, 1999).
Cultural

Gender Roles and Violence as Conflict Resolution

At the societal level, violence against women is most common where gender roles are rigidly defined and enforced (Heise, 1998) and where the concept of masculinity is linked to toughness, male honor, or dominance (Counts et al., 1992). Other cultural norms associated with IPV include acceptance of violence as a means to settle interpersonal disagreements and tolerance of physical punishment of women and children (Levinson, 1989). Levinson's study found that societal norms governing conflict were more strongly related to low levels of wife-beating than to a need to exhibit aggressive behavior in order to project a macho image.

Male Dominance and Masculine Ideology

Male dominance in society is characterized by the control of organizational and economic resources by men (Levinson, 1989). Societal endorsement of male dominance produces societies in which women have little or no access to political systems, participation in the economy, or influence in academic life or the arts. In addition, patriarchal societies tend not to take violence against women seriously, as reflected in their laws, criminal justice system operations, and police attitudes. Related to male dominance is the perception that men have "ownership" of women (Heise, 1998; Levinson; Orpinas, 1999).

"Hypermasculinity," "hostile masculinity," and "patriarchal ideology" are constructs of male gender identity that have been related to increased likelihood of perpetrating violence against women. Hypermasculine men have internalized to an extreme degree those cultural messages that equate manliness with fearlessness, toughness, and risk-taking. Certain male peer groups, such as gangs, campus fraternities, intercollegiate or professional team sports, and military units, are particularly adept at reinforcing the macho script through such behaviors as thrill-seeking, fighting, and bragging about sexual conquests. Mosher and colleagues (Mosher & Anderson, 1986; Mosher & Sirkin, 1984; Mosher & Tomkins, 1988) found that men who rated high on hypermasculinity were more likely to report perpetrating sexual aggression against women. Mosher and Tomkins used script theory to explain that hypermasculine men would be more prone to use sexual coercion against women because the show of forcefulness, domination, and danger involved validates their masculinity.

Hostile masculinity, as described by Malamuth, Scokloski, Koss, and Tanaka (1991), consists of a desire to be in control, to be dominant (particularly in sexual relationships with women), and to be distrustful of women. Hostile masculinity is also related to hostility toward and an acceptance of violence against women (Malamuth & Thornhill, 1994). Hostile masculinity may lead to sexual aggression through endorsement of rape myths, adversarial sexual beliefs, and sexual promiscuity, which in interaction with hostility can produce sexual assault (Malamuth, 1996; Malamuth et al.).

A meta-analysis by Sugarman and Frankel (1996) defined patriarchal ideology in terms of measures of attitudes toward violence, conservative attitudes toward gender-roles, and gender-role traits. In examining the predicted relationship between wife assault and maintenance of patriarchal ideology in 29 studies, they found that attitudes toward violence predicted IPV most strongly ($d = .71$); the relationship between attitudes toward gender roles were less strongly predictive ($d = .54$). Strong endorsement of masculine gender role was not associated with IPV; in fact, the effect was not in the predicted direction ($d = -.14$), although this last finding was based on only four studies.

Murnen, Wright, and Kaluzny (2002) conducted a meta-analysis of 39 studies that related masculine ideology to violence against women, specifically sexual aggression. Masculine ideology was measured in terms of attitudes toward violence and dominance in general, attitudes toward women, attitude toward violence in relationships with women, and gender role adherence measures. They found that the two largest effects were for hypermasculinity (d = .61) and hostile masculinity (d = .58), both of which measure multiple components of masculine ideology (acceptance of aggression against women and negative and hostile beliefs about women). The next strongest relationships were male dominance over women (d = .56) and measures of hostility toward women (d = .54). Gender role traits, as measured by gender role stereotyping and masculine instrumentality, were not strongly predictive of sexual violence. While these findings support a sociocultural model that uses acceptance of patriarchal ideology to predict sexual aggression, the authors caution against inferring that possession of patriarchal attitudes toward women is sufficient to perpetuate sexual aggression. Situational characteristics, such as heavy alcohol consumption, peer pressure, or lack of social conscience and irresponsibility, may also need to be present for coercive sexual encounters to occur.

Religious Conservatism

Conventional wisdom suggests that because members of certain types of religious denominations (e.g., fundamentalist) tend to endorse primacy of male authority in the home, they may be more likely to condone a husband's right to control his wife through violence (Heggen, 1996; Singh & Unnithan, 1999; Walker, 1999). Ellison, Bartowski, and Anderson (1999) examined data from a national probability sample of 13,017 men and women ages 18 and older to test this hypothesis, and to investigate whether sharing the same denomination and frequency of church attendance decreased the likelihood of IPV. Researchers found that men who held more conservative theological views than their female partners, regardless of whether they were of the same conservative denomination, were more likely to perpetrate IPV.

Intervention Strategies

By combining individual-level risk factors with findings of cross-cultural studies, it can easily be seen how an ecological model such as the one proposed by Heise (1998) and Jewkes (2002) contributes to the understanding of why some societies and some individuals are more violent than others, and why women, especially wives, are so consistently the victims of abuse. Table 1 depicts the various factors that would make up such an ecological model.

Such an integrated model is sorely needed. A report by the Committee on Assessment of Family Violence Intervention of the Institute of Medicine and the National Research Council (Chalk & King, 1998) noted that while billions of dollars were spent each year to curb family violence, most treatment and intervention efforts supported by these funds were created in the absence of solid scientific evidence. Further, few programs were evaluated for their effectiveness. The committee found that in many communities, healthcare, social service agencies, and law enforcement interventions exist alongside one another in an uncoordinated system, which is for the most part undocumented and poorly understood. Only 114 studies conducted from 1980 to 1996 had sufficient scientific strength to allow inferences to be drawn about the effects of specific interventions for family violence (Chalk & King). Most studies evaluated social service programs for child maltreatment, not IPV, and only a few evaluated interventions in the health care setting.

Wathen and MacMillan (2003) recently completed a systematic review of the scientific literature on interventions for violence against women. In addition to conducting a thorough and extensive search for relevant studies, the authors applied the rigorous standards of the Canadian Task Force on Preventive Health Care to rate the quality of each study. Since the purpose of the review was to provide primary health care providers with evidence-based strategies to prevent abuse or re-abuse for patients identified as IPV victims, the authors focused on secondary, rather than primary, prevention efforts targeting factors at the individual and interpersonal levels of the social ecological model. The results of their assessment are used to document empirical evidence for secondary prevention efforts aimed at the inner two layers of the model. However, I have expanded their criteria to include primary prevention programs that have some evidence indicating effectiveness. Because this paper focuses on programs that address all levels of the social ecological model, I have also included promising primary and secondary prevention strategies that address factors at the outer layers of the model, even though they may not have been evaluated. Table 2 displays a summary of the intervention strategies discussed that address factors at these two levels of the ecological model.

TABLE 1. Factors Within Each Level of an Ecological Model of IPV (adapted from Heise, 1998; Jewkes, 2002)

Personal History	Interpersonal	Community	Culture
Gender: males more likely to be batterers, females more likely to be victims	Male control of wealth and decision-making in the family	Poverty, low economic status, unemployment	Norms granting males control over female behavior
Being abused and/or witnessing violence between parents during childhood	Marital conflict	Isolation of women and family	Acceptance of violence as a means of resolving conflict
Education of women; female empowerment	Alcohol Use	Male peer groups that condone violence against women	Notion of masculinity linked to dominance, aggression, honor
Male hostility towards women			Rigid gender roles

PRIMARY PREVENTION

Individual Level

Family visitation programs to prevent early childhood abuse and witnessing of IPV. A systematic review of published studies (Anderson, Shinn, & St. Charles, 2002) was conducted by a team of experts to determine the effectiveness of programs designed to reduce child maltreatment. Child maltreatment was defined as witnessing IPV or experiencing abuse and/or neglect in childhood, all of which are risk factors for experiencing or perpetrating violence as an adult. The priority population for these intervention programs were families considered to be at high risk of child maltreatment: single or young mothers, low-income households, and families with low birth weight infants (Anderson et al.).

Home visitation coupled with parental training programs was examined. Overall, home visitation programs resulted in a 40% reduction in child maltreatment episodes. To be effective, visits needed to occur during at least part of the child's first two years of life, though they may have been initiated during pregnancy and may have continued after the child's second birthday. Programs of longer duration had better outcomes; in general, programs of less than two years duration were not effective. Professional home visitors appeared to be more effective than trained paraprofessionals, but longer-duration programs with trained paraprofessionals were also found to be effective (Anderson et al., 2002). While these programs appeared to be effective in reducing child

TABLE 2. Intervention Strategies to Address Factors at Each Level of the Ecological Model

	Individual Level	Interpersonal Level	Community Level	Cultural Level
Primary Prevention	Family visitation programs and parental training	Youth dating violence prevention	Worksite violence prevention	Structural and policy supports "Men's work" Public health social marketing activities
Secondary Prevention	Screening in health care settings and emergency departments Prenatal screening & counseling Advocacy, shelter stays, and counseling Batterer treatment	Couples counseling and family therapy	Law enforcement IPV protocols and protection orders Legal advocacy for victims	

maltreatment, there was insufficient evidence to draw conclusions about the impact of visiting programs on other types of violence such as IPV. However, given the strong and consistent link between experiencing or witnessing family violence in childhood and future perpetration/victimization, these programs seem promising as primary prevention strategies.

Interpersonal: Couples, Families, and Neighbors

Adolescent dating violence. Adolescence is an opportune time for primary prevention of IPV. For some, it marks the bridge between childhood maltreatment and the perpetuation of the cycle of violence within their own adult relationships (Wekerle & Wolfe, 1999; Wolfe & Jaffe, 1999). Adolescents who have had inconsistent, authoritarian, or neglectful parenting may lack experience in healthy relationships, and be more likely to have power-based expectations for their own and their partner's behavior as they begin dating (Wekerle & Wolfe). Some researchers have suggested that abusive behavior in adolescence can be experimental in nature, less firmly tied to gender role expectations, and more amenable to influence and change (e.g., Moffitt, 2004). In either case, adolescent dating programs can help adolescents transition from self-focused, dependent childhood relationships to more reciprocal, equality-based relationships as they grow into adulthood (Wekerle & Wolfe).

While the dynamics of adolescent dating violence are poorly understood, prevalence studies indicate that between 10-25% of high school students and 20-30% of college students have experienced relationship violence (Wekerle & Wolfe, 1999). Unlike violence between adult partners, adolescent dating violence appears to be less dependent on gender. Studies indicate that girls are equally as likely to perpetrate physical and emotional abuse as boys (Avery-Leaf, Cascardi, O'Leary, & Cano, 1997; Cascardi, Avery-Leaf, O'Leary, & Smith Slep, 1999; Foshee, Linder, MacDougall, & Bangdiwala, 2001; Spencer & Bryant, 2000). A review of adolescent dating violence prevention programs was conducted in the late 1990s (Wekerle & Wolfe). The review included four school-based programs (Avery-Leaf et al.; Hammond & Yung, 1991; Jaffe, Sudermann, Reitzel, & Killip, 1992; Lavoie, Vezina, Piche, & Boivin, 1995), one community based program (Wolfe et al., 1996), and one that combined school and community approaches (Foshee et al., 1996). All programs reported significant outcomes, including changes in attitudes towards IPV, knowledge of myths about violence against women, and intentions regarding constructive responses to hypothetical conflict situations. Two studies also showed a reduction in self-reported perpetration of dating violence (Foshee et al.; Wolfe et al.), although the impact of the program on self-reported victimization rates was unclear. Wekerle and Wolfe concluded that findings should be considered preliminary due to limited follow-up and generalizability.

Community: Institutions and Social Structures

Worksite violence prevention. California Department of Industrial Relations Division of Occupational Safety and Health (1995) categorized workplace violence into three types: (a) those perpetrated by unknown assailants or those who have no legitimate relationship to the workplace, (b) those involving violent interactions between customers/clients and workers, and (c) assaults between current or former co-workers or between co-workers and managers. Peek-Asa, Howard, Vargas, and Kraus, (1997) included a fourth type: perpetration of violence by personal acquaintances of an employee/customer who are neither customers or employees themselves. Workplace incidents involving IPV would fall into this fourth category.

Runyan, Zakocs, and Zwerling (2000) conducted a critical review of the literature on administrative and behavioral interventions for workplace violence. Their search of 17 databases yielded 137 papers, 41 of which described intervention strategies. Of these 41, only 9 included a program evaluation. While none of the 41 papers described workplace intervention programs focused specifically on IPV, many of the strategies could be adapted to address violence perpetrated by intimate partners. The impact of IPV in the workplace goes beyond acts of violence perpetrated on site. Victims of IPV affect productivity through absenteeism related to injuries as well as "presenteeism" (workers are on the job but have impaired productivity due to physical and psychological trauma). Thus, the existence of an Employee Assistance Program as part of an overall strategy to reduce violence perpetrated by angry or frustrated employees can be a useful entry point for abused employees to access social services for IPV. Workplace violence involving employees who are battered differs from other types of violence in that often the assailant is known to management and fellow workers, and therefore not perceived as a threat. Thus, educational programs about the dynamics of IPV can raise awareness, encourage social support, and promote peer-intervention for victims of IPV. Finally, a well designed violence prevention program in the workplace can help change social norms by causing people to question the acceptability of violence as a means to resolve conflicts.

Cultural

Structural and policy supports. Along with establishment of women's shelters and batterer treatment programs, changes in law enforcement policy and criminal justice practice have been the primary focus of IPV prevention efforts in the U.S., lifting it out of the private, domestic sphere and setting it squarely into the public domain as a human rights issue (Mills, 1996). Legal interventions include prosecuting batterers, imposing mandatory arrest laws, reforming police procedures, and issuing protective orders. In the U.S., legal interventions have met with limited success. Some research shows a decline in the number of women victimized by an intimate partner (Bureau of Justice Statistics, 2000). On the other hand, arrest and prosecution may only produce a short term reduction in battering by minor offenders, with the additional potential of escalating violence by more serious offenders in the long run (Pate & Hamilton, 1992). Civil protection orders, which require the batterer to refrain from further violence and threats, may be effective but only if they are of sufficient duration and are routinely enforced by law enforcement (Holt, Kernic, Lumley, Wolf, & Rivara, 2002). Legal and policy initiatives have an effect beyond immediate control of IPV. Some researchers believe that "people take their cues regarding the seriousness of behavior from the criminal justice system and that laws reflect emerging social norms" (Hingson & Howland, 1989, as paraphrased by Salazar, Baker, Price, & Carlin, 2003, p. 254). Policy is thought to influence behavior through two mechanisms: deterrence and social influence (Cialdini, 1995; Friedkin, 2001; Stark, 1993; Zimring & Hawkins, 1973). Salazar et al. sought to determine whether criminal justice policies on domestic violence, as perceived by the public, had an impact on social norms. They found that those who perceive that the criminal justice system actively intervened (by arresting, prosecution, sentencing, etc.) tended to be supportive of these interventions. Respondents who believed criminal justice system responses were appropriate were also less likely to hold women responsible for the abuse. The authors suggest that the impact of policies on social norms is most likely an iterative process; as social norms shift enough to permit advocacy for changes in law enforcement practice, judicial response, and judicial disposition, new IPV policies come into being. In turn, these policies shift perceptions and social norms of the wider population. When policies fail to affect social norms, however, policy is less likely to be enforced and fails over time. For this reason, the authors strongly suggest that educational campaigns targeting both social system personnel and the general public accompany newly enacted policies in order to strengthen their impact on prevailing norms.

Other policy initiatives have been implemented by national, state, and local governments worldwide. Examples include educational campaigns (Montano, 1992), task force and commission reports (Australian Law Reform Commission, 1993; Canadian Panel on Violence Against Women, 1993), constitutional amendments (Brazilian Constitution, 1988), and other law reforms. What causes some governments to implement policies and programs to combat IPV while others do not? Weldon (2002) examined social factors thought to be associated with policies that address violence against women in 36 democratic countries over a 20-year period. Contrary to her expectations, she found that neither economic level, religion, region, the number of women, nor the presence of women in government predicted governmental responsiveness to violence against women. Rather, it was the presence of a strong, active, influential, and independently organized women's movement that determined whether violence against women appeared on the public agenda. In addition, the breadth and scope of governmental response was greatly enhanced by the presence of an office dedicated to promoting women's rights (Weldon).

There are several international efforts that seek to systematically change existing social and cultural norms and frame violence against women as a human rights issue, thereby setting a global standard of justice that extends to public treatment of women as well as their treatment in the home. These efforts include the Beijing Platform for Action, the Convention for the Elimination of Discrimination Against Women, and Amnesty International. In addition, the United Nations (2004) established the Development Fund for Women (UNIFEM), whose primary concern is the status of women. UNIFEM-funded programs use culturally-relevant strategies to improve the status of women through education, empowerment, and promotion of active participation in public life. While UNIFEM supports programs that address violence against women in general and IPV specifically, many of its programs directly address the root causes of abuse: women's poverty, exclusion from the political process, lack of education, and second-class status in society.

Men's work. A number of programs have been designed to change social norms regarding male gender roles. For example, Heise (1998) describes the "Harnessing Self Reliant Initiatives and Knowledge" program in the Philippines that uses gender training as a starting point for men to organize against violence in depressed areas of Quezon City. Another group called "Support for Women Advocates of Talanay" was formed to help men become aware of gender issues. Members of the group intervene with the abusive husbands of women who have sought help at the local crisis center (Heise). A significant increase in violent crimes prompted the Men's Committee of the Icelandic Equal Rights Council to create a week-long information educational program, "Men Against Violence," that included an art exhibit, lectures on family violence, referrals to community resources for treatment, pamphlets for students at secondary schools, and a mass media campaign (Kunz, 1996).

The Family Violence Prevention Fund (FVPF) initiated a campaign in the U.S. called "Coaching Boys into Men" that encouraged adult males, acting within their roles as fathers, brothers, coaches, teachers, uncles, and mentors, to engage boys in conversations about how they treat other boys and women (FVPF, n.d.). The "Coaching Boys into Men" campaign consisted of public service announcements developed by the FVPF and The Advertising Council that encouraged men to get involved and offered strategies for talking to boys about domestic violence. The key prevention strategy promoted in the campaign is encouraging men to have conversations about domestic violence with the boy(s) in their lives, within an overall context of a trusting relationship. Men are encouraged to teach children from an early age that violence is not an acceptable way to express anger and frustration, and to serve as role models for boys by manifesting non-violent behavior in their own intimate relationships and sharing personal experiences in which they handled anger, frustration, and interpersonal conflict in constructive and non-violent ways (FVPF, n.d.).

The Oakland Men's Project (OMP) is one of the oldest community-based violence prevention organizations in the U.S. (Kivel, 1992). The OMP employs a workshop format, named "Men's Work," to eliminate men's violence by changing men's beliefs, attitudes, and skills. Workshops encourage men to explore racism, sexism, sexual harassment, and heterosexism as underlying causes of men's violence and provide them with strategies they need to resist, prevent, and change violent and abusive situations. OMP also conducts in-school and community-based youth programs that provide violence prevention skills training and cultural awareness (Kivel).

Hong (2000) presented qualitative data from a year-long case study of a men's peer education organization (Men Against Violence, or MAV) at a large university in a southern state in the U.S. This study focused on a group of eight male student organizational board officers to assess the extent to which participating in MAV changed their concepts of masculinity and attitudes toward violence during their 9- to 12-month tenure. Findings were organized according to aspects of traditional hegemonic masculinity described by Brannon and David (1976): "no sissy stuff," "be a big wheel," "be a sturdy oak," and "give 'em hell." While Hong observed some superficial qualitative changes in knowledge and attitudes in this group of men, traditional concepts and concerns persisted at a deeper level. Hong also detected a strong homophobic undercurrent. He noticed that MAV officers frequently boasted about their heterosexual exploits and engaged in homophobic behavior ("no sissy stuff"). While many in the sample endorsed attitudes against IPV and sexual assault, the concept of diffusing a conflict involving other men before it escalated to physical violence was difficult for them to accept. Most felt obligated to respond to perceived slights to their manhood by other men ("give 'em hell"), and especially felt it wrong not to physically retaliate if another man tried to intimidate or hit them. Perhaps the biggest attitudinal change in this sample occurred in their reformulation of the masculine tenet of emotional self-sufficiency ("be a sturdy oak"). Through working together, conducting educational programs, and participating in weekly "rap sessions," these men developed new insights about relationships and developed skills to build and sustain intimate friendships with other men (Hong). These findings suggest that results of socialization to hegemonic masculinity is deeply internalized in most men and not easily undone, although programs such as MAV may somewhat change men's attitudes toward gender norms and violence.

Public health social marketing activities. Currently, public health education campaigns seek to raise awareness, change attitudes, and promote behavior change with regard to a health issue. A campaign may be based on the Theory of Reasoned Action, which states that an individual's beliefs about social norms and expectations influence his/her intention to act (Ajzen & Fishbein, 1980). Knowledge about the importance of IPV as a social problem is not sufficient; the public must also perceive it to be socially acceptable to speak up about the issue to family and friends and to offer help to a victim or to expose a perpetrator. Another theory used is the Health Belief Model, which states an individual's decision to take action depends on his/her perceptions of the risk, consequences, and costs associated with taking action (Becker, 1974; Rosenstock, 1974). People usually take action only when they perceive a health risk to be severe. Social Cognitive Theory (Bandura, 1986, 1992) suggests that an individual must possess the skills necessary to perform a desired behavior, and must also believe that s/he possesses the ability to use those skills. By using people with whom a target audience can identify to model behavior, information is provided on how to do something, and the message conveyed is "if the average person can do this, so can I."

In the early 1990s, the FVPF, a national organization based in San Francisco, California, launched a new initiative, "There's No Excuse for Domestic Violence" (Klein, Campbell, Soler, & Ghez, 1997; Marin, Zia, & Soler, 1998). Formative research revealed that people already had a high level of awareness of IPV and many were personally acquainted with victims, yet still took no action. Barriers to action included a complex web of factors: a lack of social permission for intervention, a set of beliefs that minimized the severity of the problem, and a lack of self-efficacy or a sense that the average person lacked the necessary skills to successfully intervene. Thus, the campaign's central marketing message was that people not only have a right to get involved in violence intervention, but society also expects them to. Program evaluation indicated that the campaign's greatest impact on public attitudes occurred in markets with heavy media exposure: people were more likely to recall campaign messages, to perceive IPV as an important public issue, and believe that perpetrators should be held accountable by the criminal justice system. In addition, there was an increase in the number of people who reported they had recently taken action against IPV (Klein et al.).

Other campaigns have been more rigorously evaluated. Gadomski, Tripp, Wolff, Lewis, and Jenkins (2001)) measured the impact of a public health campaign targeting attitudes towards IPV in a rural county. Statistically significant increases in slogan and advertising recognition occurred in the intervention county, particularly among men recalling the campaign slogan, and in the percentage of respondents who thought that most people should talk to the victim, consult with friends, or talk to a doctor. In addition, calls to the local women's advocacy center hotline in the intervention county doubled following the campaign (Gadomski et al.).

SECONDARY PREVENTION

Individual Level

Screening in health care settings and emergency departments. Physicians generally have a two-part strategy with regard to IPV: (a) screening patients to ascertain whether they are currently being abused or are at risk of being abused, and (b) referring abused individuals (and their partners) to intervention programs and community resources. A number of screening tools (including screenings for pregnant women) have been shown to be accurate in detecting abuse (Attala, Hudson, & McSweeney, 1994; Feldhaus et al., 1997; Hegarty, Sheehan, & Schonfeld, 1999; Hudson & McIntosh, 1981; Kozoil-McLain, Coates, & Lowenstein, 2001; Rodenburg & Fantuzzo, 1993; Shepard & Campbell, 1992; Straus, Hamby, Boney-McCoy, & Sugarman, 1996; Tolman, 1999). However, Wathen and MacMillan (2003) found no studies using a comparative design that evaluated the effectiveness of different screening tools in terms of improved outcomes. For this reason, the authors focused on the use of referral resources by abused women identified through screening in healthcare settings. Referral options included finding a safe place for abused women, counseling, community based resources for women, and referral of male abusers to batterers treatment.

Due to the high prevalence of annual and lifetime experience of IPV among women who present to an emergency department (ED; Chalk & King, 1998), a number of EDs have implemented protocols for IPV assessment and intervention. In New Zealand, Fanslow, Norton, Robinson, and Spinola (1998) developed and tested a protocol based on the principles of care outlined by the American Medical Association (1992). The authors reported that immediately after IPV staff training and implementation of the protocol, a higher number of confirmed (as opposed to suspected) IPV cases were recorded, and documentation of abuse improved. Victims of IPV were also offered more treatment options. However, these improvements were not sustained at 1-year follow-up. In their review of IPV assessment and intervention training programs for ED staff, Wathen and MacMillan (2003) concluded that this approach may indeed improve the identification of and response to violence against women. However, further research is required to substantiate the link between identification of abuse and long-term outcomes.

Prenatal screening and counseling. McFarlane, Parker, Soeken, and Bullock (1992) screened pregnant women for the presence of abuse at a prenatal clinic, and found that 17% reported physical or sexual abuse, more than double the percentage range shown in previous research. McFarlane, Soeken, Reel, Parker, and Silva (1997) examined a sample of pregnant, mostly Hispanic women who had experienced IPV in a quasi-randomized design to investigate three levels of intervention: (a) an information card, (b) professional counseling, and (c) counseling combined with outreach by a peer mentor. Severe abuse decreased in all three groups, though no statistically significant differences were observed between groups at 18-month follow-up.

Advocacy, shelter stays, and/or counseling. Sullivan and colleagues (Sullivan & Bybee, 1999; Sullivan, Campbell, Angelique, Eby, & Davidson, 1994; Sullivan & Davidson, 1991) randomly assigned 284 abused women to either 10 weeks of advocacy services at 4-6 hours per week or to no contact. The intervention group reported less abuse, less physical violence, and better quality of life at the two-year follow-up, although there were no differences in reported psychological abuse or depression. To evaluate the effectiveness of shelter stays, Berk, Newton, and Berk (1986) compared a cohort of 57 women who had a shelter stay with 98 abused women who did not stay in a shelter. The study showed that 81% of women in the study reported no new violence regardless of shelter status.

Cox and Stoltenberg (1991) evaluated a program of personal and vocational counseling for women who were in protective services, and found that those who were in counseling for at least two weeks showed some improvements in self-esteem; however, the small sample size and high drop out rate made it hard to draw conclusions about the overall effectiveness of this approach.

Batterer's treatment. In the late 1980s, a rapid growth in pro-arrest policies for domestic violence prompted courts to begin mandating counseling for male offenders as a means of dealing with overloaded court dockets and as an alternative to incarceration; it was also hoped that court-mandated counseling would add a rehabilitative component to the deterrent effects of arrest (Malloy, McCloskey, & Monford, 1999). Early evaluation studies of batterer treatment programs showed promising results in lowering the frequency and severity of re-abuse. Upon critical appraisal, however, the success found in these studies appeared to be more an artifact of poor evaluation methods rather than a true reflection of program effectiveness (Gondolf, 1987; Hanmer & Griffiths, 2000; Paymar, 1993; Paymar & Pence, 1993).

Ford and Regoli (1993) examined the effects of different criminal justice approaches to 678 batterers charged with IPV over a 13 month period by randomly assigning them to one of three groups: (a) pretrial diversion to a batterer's treatment program, (b) conviction with a mandated referral to a batterer's treatment program as a condition of probation, or (c) recommendation of presumptive sentencing that did not include batterer's treatment. At six months post-adjudication, the authors found no significant differences in the rate of re-assault for any of the three groups. Dunford (2000) reported the results of a randomized controlled trial involving married U.S. Navy couples, in which the active duty husband had a history of substantiated wife abuse. Couples were randomly placed into four 12-month intervention groups: (a) group sessions for men employing a cognitive-behavioral approach, (b) conjoint group sessions for men and their wives, (c) rigorous monitoring and monthly individual counseling for men, and (d) a control group. No statistically significant differences were found across the four groups for prevalence of new or continued IPV, or time to recidivism. Feder and Dugan (2002) randomly assigned all male IPV defendants to either one year probation with court-mandated counseling or one year probation. Victim reports, batterer self-reports, and official records of re-arrest were used to determine recidivism at one year follow-up. No significant differences between the experimental and control group were found for re-arrest rates or in rates of minor and severe IPV. In addition, there were no differences in attitude, beliefs, and behaviors between the two groups. Feder and Dugan did find that variables associated with a stake in conformity (e.g., employment, age) predicted both treatment compliance and recidivism.

On the other hand, Taylor, Davis, and Maxwell (2001) used official records, victim reports, and batter self-reports to measure recidivism, and found that men in a 26-week program had fewer incidents of violence (10%) than those in a short-term (25%) or control group (26%). Palmer, Brown, and Barrera (1992) also found significantly lower rates of physical violence in a treatment group (10%) compared to a control group (31%) based on police records at 12 month follow-up. Thus, results concerning the effectiveness of batterer treatment continue to be mixed.

Interpersonal Level

Couples, families, and neighbors. While Wathen and MacMillan (2003) found some evidence to support the effectiveness of couples therapy as an IPV intervention, these types of studies tend to be of poor or fair methodological quality. The San Diego Navy Experiment (Dunford, 2000), which employed a rigorous random controlled trial design, did not find couples counseling to be effective in reducing IPV. Couples counseling is usually not the preferred level of immediate intervention due to a heightened risk of further violence (Deschner, 1984). Once the violence has stopped, couples counseling and family therapy may be used.

One concern expressed by IPV advocates is that the use of couples' counseling based on systems theory ignores the obvious power inequality between partners, implying that each carry responsibility for the abuse. On the other hand, Goldner (1998) argues that couples treatment may be modified to address individual trauma, safety, and relationship issues while taking a clear moral position that violence is unacceptable in any form. Goldner also states that couples' counseling may reinforce the social unacceptability of violence: "...the victim speaking her experience to her abusive partner in the presence of concerned others...who are "bearing witness" creates a moral imperative that...[makes] the man's accountability all the more real" (p. 265).

Community Level

Law enforcement protocols for handling IPV at the scene. Sherman and Berk (1984) evaluated the Minneapolis Domestic Violence Experiment, in which police implemented three randomly assigned protocols: (a) arrest the perpetrator, (b) separate the couple, or (c) provide advice. At six months, violent recidivism was markedly lower for the group of perpetrators who were arrested compared to the other two groups. This study led to the arrest of the perpetrator at the scene as the preferred police strategy for IPV, as well as a shift in the definition of IPV as personal family problem to IPV as a crime. Six replication studies (Garner, Fagan, & Maxwell, 1995) found variable results in the effectiveness of police arrest policies, however. While some duplicated the results of the Minneapolis study, others showed an escalation of violence among males who were arrested. These findings led to an awareness of the interaction between individual characteristics of the perpetrator, the correct implementation of the arrest policies by law enforcement, the importance of cross-jurisdictional buy-in, and effectiveness of arrest. Arrest appeared to have a stronger affect on employed men compared to unemployed men, the rationale being that employed men had more to lose if arrested (Pate & Hamilton, 1992). Unfortunately, correct implementation of the new arrest policies by jurisdiction was not evaluated when comparing outcomes, but it was known to have varied.

Researchers found that women who obtained protection orders of 12 months' duration had an 80% decrease in reported incidence of physical violence in the year following the intervention compared to women who had no protective order (Holt et al., 2002). On the other hand, no difference in subsequent reported physical abuse was found for women who obtained two-week civil protection orders compared to a reference group. Moreover, protection orders were associated with an increase in psychological abuse. Again, enforcement of these protection orders by police was not examined, and the effects of varying enforcement levels are unknown.

Legal advocates for women. Few studies examine the outcomes of advocacy for battered women. Bell and Goodman (2001) employed a quasi-random design to compare women assigned to advocacy services that included legal representation and support, referral to community agencies, information about IPV, and other instrumental social support to a comparison group. They found less psychological and physical re-abuse in the intervention group. Despite the non-standard randomization procedure, high attrition at follow-up, and small sample size, these promising results warrant further study (Wathen & MacMillan 2003).

Koss' (2000) assessment of the adversarial criminal justice response is that it is largely ineffective in preventing further violence by IPV perpetrators, and is fundamentally unfair because it puts the burden of proof on the victim and may result in re-traumatization. Some IPV experts have suggested that the retributive justice model currently used be replaced or supplemented with *restorative justice* approaches (van Wormer & Bednar, 2002). Restorative justice, which seeks to involve victims in the justice process and address the harm done to them, includes (a) civil proceedings, (b) victim-offender reparation through mediation, and (c) "communitarian approaches" (see below). It should be noted, however, that the civil justice system has the same shortcomings as the criminal justice system, where conflict mediation is predicated on the assumption that each party has both equal personal power and equal responsibility for the violence.

For these reasons, Koss (2000) and others see communitarian justice as a promising approach. The basic principle of communitarian justice is simple: "In the wake of an offense, and where guilt is admitted, victims, offenders, and their supporters are given an opportunity to meet in the presence of a coordinator or facilitator...encouraged to discus the direct or indirect effects of the incident on them...[and to] negotiate plans for repairing the damage and minimizing further harm" (p. 1337). Forms of communitarian justice have been practiced in indigenous societies and have been used in the U.S. to resolve cases of juvenile justice, drunk driving, and IPV among the Navajo (Koss). Koss and colleagues have also described application of this model with victims of sexual assault in Pima County, Arizona (Koss, Bachar, & Hopkins, 2003). Outcomes research on the effectiveness of this promising approach is eagerly awaited.

Implications and Future Directions

This paper has reviewed studies that investigate factors at various levels of the ecological IPV model described by Heise (1998). Some factors, such as the relationship between childhood abuse and future victimization, have been the subject of a number of studies that employed strong research designs and thus enjoy firm empirical support for their predictive role in IPV. Other factors, such as female empowerment via education, employment, and income, have been studied less frequently. In addition, only a few studies have employed multilevel study designs to examine the impact of contextual factors on individual characteristics (e.g., Cunradi et al., 2000; Hinden & Adair, 2002; Koenig et al., 2003). More multilevel epidemiologic studies of causal influences are needed to better understand the mechanisms by which complex factors such as gender roles, poverty, and cultural norms interact to produce IPV.

This paper has attempted to describe existing intervention studies that address risk factors at various levels of the model. The majority of interventions reviewed involves secondary prevention and focus on the individual, such as identification of victims, referral to victim services, and sanctions and/or treatment programs for batterers. Some of the more familiar interventions, such as batterer's treatment programs and arrest protocols, have been relatively well studied. Others have been studied only minimally (e.g., screening programs for victims in health care settings) or have conflicting evidence of efficacy (e.g., use of battered women's shelters and advocacy services). In addition, promising interventions that address community and cultural factors have been presented even though many of these, such as worksite violence prevention programs or "men's work" programs, have not been evaluated. Still others, such as public education campaigns and widespread policy changes, have been evaluated minimally or with poor research methods. Evaluations that employ rigorous design criteria are needed to validate the efficacy and generalizability of these promising approaches.

Jewkes (2002) proposed a number of potential primary intervention strategies not discussed in this paper due to a lack of research concerning their current use in IPV prevention programs. These include: community action theater to educate, inform, and stimulate change in attitudes; programs to empower women through education, employment, and access to micro-credit schemes; increased local and national involvement of women in political activities; and measures to reduce objectification of women in pornography and beauty pageants. These strategies, as well as others that specifically target men, should be implemented as part of community based intervention efforts, accompanied by evaluation studies that measure their effectiveness.

REFERENCES

Abrahams, N., Jewkes, R., & Laubscher, R. (1999). *I don't believe in democracy in the home: Men's relationships with and abuse of women.* Cape Town, South Africa: MRC Technical Report.

American Medical Association. (1992). Violence against women: Relevance for medical practitioners. *Journal of the American Medical Association, 267,* 3184-3189.

Anderson, K. (1997). Gender, status, and domestic violence: An integration of feminist and family violence approaches. *Journal of Marriage and the Family, 59,* 655-680.

Anderson, L.M., Shinn, C., & St. Charles, J. (2002). Community interventions to promote healthy social environments: Early childhood development and family housing. *Morbidity and Mortality Weekly Report, Recommendations and Reports, 51*(RR01), 1-8.

Attala, J. M., Hudson, W. W., & McSweeney, M. (1994). A partial validation of two short-form Partner Abuse Scales. *Women's Health, 21*, 125-139.

Australian Law Reform Commission. (1993). *Equality before the law* (Discussion Paper 54). Sydney, Australia: Author.

Avery-Leaf, S., Cascardi, M., O'Leary, K. D., & Cano, A. (1997). Efficacy of a dating violence prevention program on attitudes justifying aggression. *Journal of Adolescent Health, 21*, 11-17.

Azjen, I., & Fishbein, M. (1980). *Understanding attitudes and predicting social behavior*. Englewood Cliffs, NJ: Prentice Hall.

Bachman, R. (2000). A comparison of annual incidence rates and contextual characteristics of intimate-partner violence against women from the National Crime Victimization Survey (NCVS) and the National Violence Against Women Survey (NVAWS). *Violence Against Women, 6, 839*-867.

Bachman, R., & Saltzman, L.E. (1995). *Violence against women: Estimates from the redesigned survey*. Washington, DC: Bureau of Justice Statistics, National Institute of Justice.

Bandura, A. J. (1986) *Social foundations of thought and action: A social cognitive theory*. Englewood Cliffs, NJ: Prentice Hall.

Bandura, A. J. (1992) Exercise of personal agency through self-efficacy mechanism. In R. Schwarzer (Ed.), *Self-efficacy: Thought control of action* (pp. 3-38). Washington, DC: Hemisphere.

Becker, M. H. (1974). The health belief model and personal health behavior. *Health Education Monographs, 2*, 324-508.

Bell, M. E., & Goodman, L. A. (2001). Supporting battered women involved with the court system: An evaluation of a law-based advocacy intervention. *Violence Against Women, 7*, 1377-1404.

Berk, R. A., Newton, P. J., & Berk, S. F. (1986). What a difference a day makes: an empirical study of the impact of shelters for battered women. *Journal of Marriage and Family, 48*, 481-490.

Bourgois, P. (1996). In search of masculinity: Violence, respect and sexuality among Puerto Rican crack dealers. *British Journal of Criminology, 36*, 412-427.

Brannon, R., & David, D. (1976). *The forty-nine percent majority: The male sex role*. Reading, MA: Addison-Wesley.

Brazilian Constitution. (1998). Art. 226, §8.

Bureau of Justice Statistics. (2000). *Criminal victimization 2000: Changes 1999-2000 with trends 1993-2000* (NCJ - 187007). Washington, DC: U.S. Government Printing Office.

Caesar, P. L. (1988). Exposure to violence in the families-of-origin among wife-abusers and maritally nonviolent men. *Violence and Victims, 3*, 49-63.

Caetano, R., Schafer, J., & Cunradi, C. B. (2001). Alcohol-related intimate partner violence among white, black, and Hispanic couples in the United States. *Alcohol Research and Health, 25*, 58-65.

California Department of Industrial Relations Division of Occupational Safety and Health (1995). *Injury and illness prevention model program for workplace security.* San Francisco, CA: Author.

Campbell, J. C. (2000). Promises and perils of surveillance in addressing violence against women. *Violence Against Women, 6,* 705-727.

Campbell, J., Jones, A. S., Dienemann, J., Kub, J., Schollenberger, J., O'Campo, P., et al. (2002). Intimate partner violence and physical health consequences. *Archives of Internal Medicine, 162,* 1157-1166.

Canadian Panel on Violence Against Women. (1993). *Changing the landscape: Ending violence, achieving equality.* Ottawa, Canada: Minister of Supply and Services.

Cascardi, M., Avery-Leaf, S., O'Leary, K. D., & Smith Slep, A. M. (1999). Factor structure and convergent validity of the Conflict Tactic Scale in high school students. *Psychological Assessment, 11,* 546-555.

Chalk, R., & King, P. (Eds.) (1998). *Violence in families: Assessing prevention and treatment programs.* Washington, DC: National Academy Press.

Cialdini, R. B. (1995). Principles and techniques of social influence. In A. Tesser (Ed.), *Advanced social psychology* (pp. 257-282). New York: McGraw Hill.

Coleman, D. H., & Straus, M. A. (1986). Marital power, conflict and violence in a nationally representative sample of American couples. *Violence and Victims, 1,* 141-157.

Connell, R. W. (1987). *Gender and power: Society, the person, and sexual politics.* Stanford, CA: Stanford University Press.

Counts, D. A., Brown, J., & Campbell, J. (Eds.) (1992). *Sanctions and sanctuary: Cultural perspectives on the beating of wives.* Boulder, CO: Westview Press.

Cox, J., & Stoltenberg, C. (1991). Evaluation of a treatment program for battered wives. *Journal of Family Violence, 6,* 395-413.

Cunradi, C.B., Caetano, R., Clark, C., & Shafer, J. (2000). Neighborhood poverty as a predictor of intimate partner violence among White, Black and Hispanic couples in the United States: A multilevel analysis. *Annals of Epidemiology, 10,* 297-308.

Cruz, J. M., & Peralta, R. L. (2001). Family violence and substance use: The perceived effects of substance use within gay male relationships. *Violence & Victims, 16,* 161-172.

DeKeseredy, W. S. (2000). Current controversies on defining nonlethal violence against women in intimate heterosexual relationships: Empirical implications. *Violence Against Women, 6,* 728-746.

Department of Health. (2003). *South Africa demographic and health survey 1998, final report.* Pretoria, South Africa: Author.

Deschner, J. (1984). *The hitting habit: Anger control for battering couples.* New York: Free Press.

Dobash, R. P., & Dobash, R. E. (1979). *Violence against wives: A case against the patriarchy.* New York: Free Press.

Dunford, F. W. (2000). The San Diego Navy experiment: An assessment of interventions for men who assault their wives. *Journal of Consulting Clinical Psychology, 68,* 468-476.

Ellison, G. C., Bartowski, J. P., & Anderson K. L. (1999). Are there religious variations in domestic violence? *Journal of Family Issues, 20,* 87-88.

Ellsberg, M. C., Pena, R., Herrera, A., Liljestrand, J., & Winkvist, A. (1999). Wife abuse among women of childbearing age in Nicaragua. *American Journal of Public Health, 89,* 241-244.

El-Zanaty, F., Hussein, E. M., Shawky, G. A., Way, A. A., & Kishor, S. (1996). *Egypt demographic and health survey, 1995.* Calverton, MD: Macro International.

Family Violence Prevention Fund. (n.d.). *Coaching boys into men.* Washington, DC: Author. Retrieved April 21, 2004 from, http://endabuse.org/cbim/

Fanslow, J. L., Norton, R. N., Robinson, E. M., & Spinola, C. G. (1998). Outcome evaluation of an emergency department protocol of care on partner abuse. *Australian New Zealand Journal of Public Health, 22,* 598-603.

Feder, L., & Dugan, L. (2002). A test of the efficacy of court-mandated counseling for domestic violence offenders: The Broward experiment. *Justice Quarterly, 19,* 343-375.

Feldhaus, K. M., Koziol-McLain, J., Amsbury, H. L., Norton, I. M., Lowenstein, S. R., & Abbott, J. T. (1997). Accuracy of 3 brief screening questions for detecting partner violence in the emergency department. *Journal of the American Medical Association, 277,* 1357-1361.

Friedkin, N. E. (2001). Norm formation in social influence networks. *Social Networks, 23,* 167-189.

Ford, D., & Regoli, M. H. (1993). The criminal prosecution of wife assaulters. In Z. Hilton (Ed.), *Legal responses to wife assault: Current trends and evaluation* (pp. 127-164). Newbury Park, CA: Sage.

Foshee, V.A., Linder, G.F., Bauman, K.E., Langwick, S.A., Arriaga, X.B., Heath, J.L., et al. (1996). The Safe Dates Project: Theoretical basis, evaluation design, and selected baseline findings. *American Journal of Preventive Medicine, 12,* 39-47.

Foshee, V. A., Linder, G. F., MacDougall, J. E. & Bangdiwala, S. (2001). Gender differences in the longitudinal predictors of adolescent dating violence. *Preventive Medicine: An International Journal Devoted to Practice and Theory, 32,* 128-141.

Gadomski, A. M., Tripp, M., Wolff, D. A., Lewis, C., & Jenkins, P. (2001). Impact of a rural domestic violence prevention campaign. *Journal of Rural Health, 17,* 266-277.

Garner, J., Fagan, J., & Maxwell, C. (1995). Published findings from the Spouse Assault Replication Program: A critical review. *Journal of Quantitative Criminology, 11,* 3-28.

Gelles, R. J. (1974). *The violent home.* Beverley Hills, CA: Sage.

Gelles, R. J. (1993). Through a sociological lens: Social structure and family violence. In R. J. Gelles & D. R. Loseke (Eds.), *Current controversies on family violence* (pp. 31-46). Newbury Park, CA: Sage.

Gelles, R. J., & Straus, M. A. (1998). *Intimate violence: the causes and consequences of abuse in the American family.* New York: Simon and Schuster.

Goldner, V. (1998). Treatment of violence and victimization in intimate relationships. *Family Process, 37,* 263-286.

Gondolf, E. (1987). *Multi-site evaluation of batterer intervention systems: Summary of the 15 month follow-up.* Minneapolis, MN: University of Minnesota. Retrieved April 1, 2004 from, http://www.minicava.umn.edu/documents/gondolf/summary/summary.shtml

Gordon, M. (2000). Definitional issues in violence against women: Surveillance and research from a violence research perspective. *Violence Against Women, 6,* 747-783.

Grigsby, N., & Hartman, B. R. (1997). The Barriers Model: An integrated strategy for intervention with battered women. *Psychotherapy: Theory, Research, Practice, Training, 34,* 485-497.

Guille, L. (2004). Men who batter and their children: An integrated review. *Aggression and Violent Behavior, 9,* 129-163.

Hammond, W. R. & Yung, B. R. (1991). Preventing violence in at-risk African-American youth. *Journal of Health Care for Poor and Underserved, 2,* 359-373

Hanmer, J., & Griffiths, S. (2000). Policing repeated domestic violence by men. In J. Hanmer & C. Ittzin (Eds.), *Home truths about domestic violence: Feminist influences on policy and practice–A reader* (pp. 323-339). London, UK: Routledge.

Hastings, J. E., & Hamberger, L. K. (1997). Sociodemographic predictors of violence. *Psychiatric Clinics of North America, 20,* 323-335.

Hegarty, K., Sheehan, M., & Schonfeld, C. (1999). A multidimensional definition of partner abuse: Development and preliminary validation of the Composite Abuse Scale. *Journal of Family Violence, 14,* 399-415.

Heggen, C. H. (1996). Religious beliefs and abuse. In C.C. Kroeger & J. R. Beck (Eds.), *Women, abuse and the Bible: How scripture can be used to hurt or to heal* (pp. 15-27). Grand Rapids, MI: Baker Books.

Heise, L. (1998). Violence against women: An integrated, ecological framework. *Violence Against Women, 4,* 262-290.

Heise, L. (2002). A global overview of gender-based violence. *International Journal of Gynecology and Obstetrics, 78* (Suppl. 1), S5-S14.

Hindin, M. J. (2000). Women's power and anthropometric status in Zimbabwe. *Social Science and Medicine. 51,* 1517-1528.

Hindin, M. J., & Adair, L. S. (2002). Who's at risk? Factors associated with intimate partner violence in the Philippines. *Social Science and Medicine, 55,* 1517-1528.

Hingson, R., & Howland, J. (1989). Alcohol, injury and legal controls: Some complex interactions. *Law, Medicine and Health Care, 19,* 58-68.

Hoffman, K. L., Demo, D. H., & Edwards, J. N. (1994). Physical wife abuse in a non-western society: An integrated theoretical approach. *Journal of Marriage and the Family, 56,* 131-146.

Holt, V. L., Kernic, M. A., Lumley, T., Wolf, M. E., & Rivara, F. P. (2002). Civil protection orders and risk of subsequent police-reported violence. *Journal of the American Medical Association, 288,* 589-594.

Hong, L. (2000). Toward a transformed approach to prevention: Breaking the link between masculinity and violence. *Journal of American College Health, 48,* 269-289.

Hornung, C. A., McCullough, B. C., & Sugimoto, T. (1981). Status relationships in marriage: Risk factors in spouse abuse. *Journal of Marriage and the Family, 43,* 675-692.

Hotaling, G. T., & Sugarman, D. B. (1986). Analysis of risk markers in husband to wife violence: The current state of knowledge. *Violence and Victims, 1,* 101-124.

Hotaling, G. T., & Sugarman, D. B. (1990). A risk marker analysis of assaulted wives. *Journal of Family Violence, 5,* 1-13.

Hudson, W. W., & McIntosh, S. R. (1981). The assessment of spouse abuse: two quantifiable dimensions. *Journal of Marriage and Family, 43*, 873-885.

International Clinical Epidemiologists Network (2000). *Domestic violence in India: A summary report of a multi-site household survey.* Washington, DC: International Center for Research on Women.

Jaffee, P. G., Sudermann, M., Reitzel, D., & Killip, S. M. (1992). An evaluation of a secondary school primary prevention program on violence in intimate relationships. *Violence and Victims, 7*, 129-146.

Jejeebhoy, S. J., & Cook, R. J. (1997). State accountability for wife-beating: The Indian challenge. *The Lancet, 349*, sI10-sI12.

Jewkes, R. (2002). Intimate partner violence: Causes and prevention. *The Lancet, 359,* 1423-1429.

Jewkes, R., Penn-Kekana, L., Levin, J. (2002). Risk factors for domestic violence: Findings from a South African cross-sectional study. *Social Science and Medicine, 55*, 1603-17.

Kalmuss, D. (1984). The intergenerational transmission of marital aggression. *Journal of Marriage and the Family, 46*, 11-19.

Kivel, P. (1992). *Men's work.* Center City, MN: Hazelden.

Klein, E., Campbell, J. C., Soler, E., & Ghez, M. (1997). *Ending domestic violence: Changing public perceptions–Halting the epidemic.* Thousand Oaks, CA: Sage.

Koenig, M. A., Ahmed, S., Hossain, M. B., & Mozumder, A. B. M. K. A. (2003). Women's status and domestic violence in rural Bangladesh: Individual and community-level effects. *Demography, 40*, 269-288.

Koss, M. P. (2000). Blame, shame, and community: Justice responses to violence against women. *American Psychologist, 55*(11), 1332-1343.

Koss, M. P., Bachar, K. J. & Hopkins, C. Q. (2003). Restorative justice for sexual violence: Repairing victims, building community and holding offenders accountable. *Annals of the New York Academy of Science, 989*, 384-396.

Koziol-McLain, J., Coates, C. J., & Lowenstein, S. R. (2001). Predictive validity of a screen for partner violence against women. *American Journal of Preventive Medicine, 21*, 93-100.

Krug, E. G., Mercy, J. A., Dahlberg, L. L., Zwi, A. B. (2002). World report on violence and health. *The Lancet, 360*, 1083-1088.

Kunz, K. (1996). Taking action against violence. *Entre Nous Copenhagen Denmark, 32*, 6-7.

Kyriacou, D.N., McCabe, F., Anglin, D., Lapesarde, K., & Winer, M.R. (1998). Emergency department-based study of risk factors for acute injury from domestic violence against women. *Annals of Emergency Medicine, 31*, 502-506.

Lavoie, F., Vezina, L., Piche, C. & Boivin, M. (1995). Evaluation of a prevention program for violence in teen dating relationships. *Journal of Interpersonal Violence, 10*, 516-524.

Leung, W. C., Leung, T. W., Lam, Y. Y., & Ho, P. C. (1999). The prevalence of domestic violence against pregnant women in a Chinese community. *International Journal of Gynaecology and Obstetrics, 66*, 23-30.

Levinson, D. (1989). *Violence in cross cultural perspective.* Newbury Park, CA: Sage.

Malamuth, N. M. (1996). *The confluence model of sexual aggression: Feminist and evolutionary perspectives.* New York: Oxford University Press.

Malamuth, N. M., Scokloski, R. J., Koss, M. P, & Tanaka, J. S. (1991). Characteristics of aggressors against women: Testing a model using a national sample of college students. *Journal of Consulting and Clinical Psychology, 59,* 670-681.

Malamuth, N. M., & Thornhill, N. W. (1994). Hostile masculinity, sexual aggression, and gender-biased domineeringness in conversations. *Aggressive Behavior, 20,* 185-293.

Malloy, K. A., McCloskey, K. A., Grigsby, N., & Gardner, D. (2003). Women's use of violence within intimate relationships. *Journal of Aggression, Maltreatment & Trauma, 6,* 37-59.

Malloy, K. A., McCloskey, K. A. & Monford, T. M. (1999). A group treatment program for male batterers. In L. Van de Creek & T. L. Jackson (Eds.), *Innovations in clinical practice: A source book* (Vol. 17, pp. 377-395). Sarasota, FL: Professional Resource Press.

Marin, L., Zia, H., & Soler, E. (1998). *Ending domestic violence: Report from the global frontlines.* San Francisco, CA: Family Violence Prevention Fund.

Martin, S. L., Tsui, A. O., Maitra, K., & Marinshaw, R. (1999). Domestic violence in Northern India. *American Journal of Epidemiology, 150,* 417-426.

McCauley, J., Kern, D. E., Kolodner, K., Dill, L., Schroeder, A. F., Dechant, H. K., et al. (1995). The "battering syndrome": Prevalence and clinical characteristics of domestic violence in primary health care internal medicine practices. *Annals of Internal Medicine, 123,* 737-746.

McFarlane, J., Parker, B., Soeken, K., & Bullock, L. (1992). Assessing for abuse during pregnancy: Severity and frequency of injuries and associated entry into prenatal care. *Journal of the American Medical Association, 267,* 3176-3178.

McFarlane, J., Soeken, K., Reel, S., Parker, B., & Silva, C. (1997). Resource use by abused women following an intervention program: Associated severity of abuse and reports of abuse ending. *Public Health Nursing, 14,* 244-250.

Mills, L. (1996). Empowering battered women: The case for postmodern interventions. *Social Work, 41,* 261-268.

Moffitt, T. E. (2004). Adolescent-limited and life-course-persistent offending: A complementary pair of developmental theories. In T. P. Thornberry (Ed), *Developmental theories of crime and delinquency* (pp. 11-54). New Brunswick, NJ: Transaction Publishers.

Montano, S. (1992). Long live the differences with equal rights: A campaign to end violence against women. In M. Schuler (Ed.), *Freedom from violence: Women's strategies from around the world* (pp. 213-226). Washington, DC: Overseas Education Fund International.

Mosher, D. L. & Anderson, R. D. (1986). Macho personality, sexual aggression, and reactions to guided imagery of realistic rape. *Journal of Research in Personality, 20,* 77-94.

Mosher. D. L., & Sirkin, M. (1984). Measuring a macho personality constellation. *Journal of Research in Personality, 18,* 150-163.

Mosher, D. L., & Tomkins, S. S. (1988). Scripting the macho man: Hypermasculine socialization and enculturation. *Journal of Sex Research, 25,* 60-84.

Murnen, S., Wright, C., & Kaluzny, G. (2002). If "boys will be boys," then will girls be victims? A meta-analytic review of the research that relates masculine ideology to sexual aggression. *Sex Roles, 46*, 359-583.

Nelson, E., & Zimmerman, C. (1996). *Household survey on domestic violence in Cambodia.* Phnom Pehn, Cambodia: Ministry of Women's Affairs and the Project Against Domestic Violence.

O'Campo, E., Gielen, A., Faden, R., Xue, X., Kass, N., & Mei-Cheng, W. (1995). Violence by male partners against women during the childbearing years: A contextual analysis. *American Journal of Public Health, 85*, 1092-1097.

Orpinas, P. (1999). Who is violent? Factors associated with aggressive behaviors in Latin America and Spain. *Pan American Journal of Public Health, 5*, 232-243.

Palmer, S. E., Brown, R. A., & Barrera, M. E. (1992). Group treatment program for abusive husbands: Long-term evaluation. *American Journal of Orthopsychiatry, 62*, 276-283.

Pate, A. M., & Hamilton, E. E. (1992). Formal and informal deterrents to domestic violence: The Dade County spouse assault experiment. *American Sociological Review, 57*, 691-697.

Paymar, M. (1993). *Violent no more: Helping men end domestic abuse.* Alameda, CA: Hunter House.

Paymar, M., & Pence, E. (1993). *Education groups for men who batter.* New York: Springer.

Peek-Asa, C., Howard, J., Vargas, L., & Kraus, J. F. (1997). Incidence of non-fatal workplace assault injuries determined from employers' reports in California. *Journal of Occupational and Environmental Medicine, 39*, 44-50.

Profamilia. (1995). *Demography and health: a survey for the socioeconomic development of the country.* Columbia: Macro International.

Rao, V. (1997). Wife-beating in rural South India: A qualitative and econometric analysis. *Social Science and Medicine, 44*, 1169-1180.

Ratner, P. A. (1993). The incidence of wife abuse and mental health status in abused wives in Edmonton, Alberta. *Canadian Journal of Public Health, 83*, 246-249.

Rodenburg, F. A., & Fantuzzo, J. (1993). The measure of wife abuse: Steps toward the development of a comprehensive assessment technique. *Journal of Family Violence, 8*, 203-227.

Rodriguez, E., Lasch, K. E., Chandra, P., & Lee, J. (2001). Family violence, employment status, welfare benefits, and alcohol drinking in the United States: What is the relation? *Journal of Epidemiology and Community Health, 55*, 172-178.

Rosenstock, I. M. (1974). The health belief model and preventive health behavior. *Health Education Monographs, 2*, 354-385.

Runyan, C. W., Zakocs, R. C., & Zwerling, C. (2000). Administrative and behavioral interventions for workplace violence prevention. *American Journal of Preventive Medicine, 18*, 116-127.

Salazar, L. F., Baker, C. K, Price, A. W., & Carlin, K. (2003). Moving beyond the individual: Examining the effects of domestic violence policies on social norms. *American Journal of Community Psychology, 32*, 253-265.

Saltzman, L. E. (2000). Building data systems for monitoring and responding to violence against women, part II. *Violence Against Women, 6*, 811-814.

Schuler, S., Hashmi, S. M., Riley, A. P., & Akhter, S. (1996). Credit programs, patriarchy and men's violence against women in rural Bangladesh. *Social Science and Medicine, 43*, 1729-1742.

Shepard, M. F., & Campbell, J. A. (1992). The abusive behavior inventory: A measure of psychological and physical abuse. *Journal of Interpersonal Violence, 7*, 291-305.

Sherman, L. W., & Berk, R. A. (1984). The specific deterrent effects of arrest for domestic assault. *American Sociological Review, 49*, 261-272.

Simons, R. L., & Johnson, C. (1998). An examination of competing explanations for the intergenerational transmission of domestic violence. In Y. Danieli (Ed.), *International handbook of multigenerational legacies of trauma* (pp. 553-570). New York: Plenum.

Singh, R. N., & Unnithan, N. P. (1999). Wife burning: Cultural cues for lethal violence against women among Asian Indians in the United States. *Violence Against Women, 5*, 641-653.

Smith, M. D. (1990). Patriarchal ideology and wife beating: A test of a feminist hypothesis. *Violence and Victims, 5*, 257-273.

South, S. J., & Spitze, G. (1994). Housework in marital and nonmarital households. *American Sociological Review, 59*, 327-347.

Spencer, G. A., & Bryant, S. A. (2000). Dating violence: A comparison of rural, suburban, and urban teens. *Journal of Adolescent Health, 27*, 302-305.

Stark, E. (1993). Mandatory arrest of batterers: A reply to its critics. *American Behavioral Scientist, 36*, 651-680.

Straus, M., & Gelles, R. J. (1990). *Physical violence in American families.* New Brunswick, NJ: Transaction Press.

Straus, M. A. (1994). State-to-state differences in social inequality and social bonds in relation to assaults on wives in the United States. *Journal of Comparative Family Studies, 25*, 7-24.

Straus, M. A., Gelles, R. J., & Steinmetz, S. K. (1980). *Behind closed doors: Violence in the American family.* New York: Anchor Press.

Straus, M. A., Hamby, S. L., Boney-McCoy, S., & Sugarman, D. B. (1996). The revised conflict tactics scales (CTS2): Development and preliminary psychometric data. *Journal of Family Issues, 17*, 283-316.

Sugarman, D. B., & Frankel, S. L. (1996). Patriarchal ideology and wife assault: A meta-analytic review. *Journal of Family Violence, 11*, 13-40.

Sullivan, C. M., & Bybee, D. I. (1999). Reducing violence using community-based advocacy for women with abusive partners. *Journal of Consulting Clinical Psychology, 67*, 43-53.

Sullivan, C. M., Campbell, R., Angelique, H., Eby, K. K., & Davidson II, W. S. (1994). An advocacy intervention program for women with abusive partners: Six-month follow-up. *American Journal of Community Psychology, 22*, 101-122.

Sullivan, C. M., & Davidson, W. (1991). The provision of advocacy services to women leaving abusive partners: An examination of short-term effects. *American Journal of Community Psychology, 19*, 953-960.

Taylor, B. G., Davis, R. C., & Maxwell, C. D. (2001). The effects of a group batterer treatment program: A randomized experiment in Brooklyn. *Justice Quarterly, 18*, 171-201.

Testa, M., & Leonard, K. E. (2001). The impact of husband physical aggression and alcohol use on marital functioning: Does alcohol "excuse" the violence? *Violence & Victims, 16*, 507-516.

Tjaden, P., & Thoennes, N. (1998). *Prevalence, incidence and consequences of violence against women: Findings from the National Violence Against Women Survey.* Washington, D.C., National Institute of Justice, Centers for Disease Control and Prevention.

Tjaden, P., & Thoennes, N. (2000a). *Extent, nature, and consequences of intimate partner violence: Findings from the National Violence Against Women Survey.* Washington, DC: US Department of Justice.

Tjaden, P., & Thoennes, N. (2000b). Prevalence and consequences of male-to-female and female-to-male intimate partner violence as measured by the National Violence Against Women Survey. *Violence Against Women, 6*, 142-161.

Tolman, R. M. (1999). The validation of the Psychological Maltreatment of Women Inventory. *Violence & Victims, 14*, 25-37.

United Nations Development Fund for Women. (2004). *About us.* Retrieved May 1, 2004 from http://www.unifem.org/index.php?f_page_pid=2

van der Straten, A., King, R., Grinstead, O., Vittinghoff, E., Serufilira, A., & Allen, S. (1998). Sexual coercion, physical violence, and HIV infection among women in steady relationships in Kigali, Rwanda. *AIDS and Behavior, 2*, 61-73.

van Wormer, K. & Bednar, S. G. (2002). Working with male batterers: A restorative strengths perspective. *Families in Society: The Journal of Contemporary Human Services, 83*(5/6), 557-565.

Vest, J. R., Catlin, T. K., Chen, J. J., & Brownson, R. C. (2002). Multistate analysis of factors associated with intimate partner violence. *American Journal of Preventive Medicine, 22*, 156-64.

Walker, L. E. (1999). Psychology and domestic violence around the world. *American Psychologist, 54*, 21-29.

Wathen, C. C., & MacMillan, H. L. (2003). Interventions for violence against women: A scientific review. *Journal of the American Medical Association, 289*, 589-600.

Watts, C., Keough, E., Ndlovu, M., & Kwaramba, R. (1998). Withholding of sex and forced sex: Dimensions of violence against Zimbabwean women. *Reproductive Health Matters. 6*, 57-65.

Wekerle, C., & Wolfe, D. A. (1999). Dating violence in mid-adolescence: Theory, significance, and emerging prevention initiatives. *Clinical Psychology Review, 19*, 435-456.

Weldon, S. L. (2002). *Protest, policy and the problem of violence against women: A cross-national comparison.* Pittsburgh, PA: University of Pittsburgh Press.

Williams, C. L. (1995). *Still a man's world.* Berkley, CA: University of California Press.

Winstock, S., Eisikovits, Z., & Gelles, R. (2002). Structure and dynamics of escalation from the batterer's perspective. *Families in Society, 83,* 129-142.

Wolfe, D. A., & Jaffe, P. G. (1999). Emerging strategies in the prevention of domestic violence. *Domestic Violence and Children, 9,* 133-144.

Wolfe, D. A., Wekerle, C., Gough, R., Reitzel-Jaffe, D., Grasley, C., Pittman, A. et al. (1996). *Youth relationships manual: A group approach with adolescents for the prevention of woman abuse and the promotion of healthy relationships.* Thousand Oaks, CA: Sage.

Zimring, R. E., & Hawkins, G. J. (1973). *Deterrence: The legal threat in crime control.* Chicago, IL: University of Chicago Press.

Submitted: January 7, 2005
Revised: January 19, 2007
Revised: May 21, 2007
Accepted: May 26, 2007

INDEX

adolescent dating violence 182-3
advocacy 24, 79, 80, 82, 89, 106,
    161, 190, 193
advocacy strategies: conduct more
    socially-responsible research
    106; identify the primary
    aggressor 107; offer appropriate
    services 107-8; outcome research
    193
African-Americans, poverty rates 14
AIDS prevention strategies 144
alcohol 36, 73, 76, 91, 96, 154, 157,
    171
Anderson, K. 175
Anglin, M. 117
Archer, J. 114
arrest: gender balance of IPV 31-4; as
    IPV prevention measure 26-7,
    31; retaliatory 35, 104; *see also*
    mandatory/preferred arrest laws
    and policies; victim arrests
arrest policies, effectiveness 193
arrest rates, women 114
Artemis Center for Alternatives to
    Domestic Violence 69, 71, 79
Asthana, S., & Oostvogels, R. 159

*Backlash: The Undeclared War
    Against Women* (Faludi) 8

battered husband syndrome: Brush on
    6; concept promotion 29
battered women: coping strategies 74,
    76; gendered expectations for 73-
    4; violence as only option for 75
batterer, identifying the primary 72-5
batterer accountability, calls for
    greater 24
batterer treatment programs: 28, 184,
    191; effectiveness 191; female
    participation 42, 88, 108
batterers, manipulation of legal
    system 35-6, 79
Bell, M. E., & Goodman, L. A. 193
Berk, R.A., Newton, P.J. & Berk, S.F.
    190
Bible A., & Osthoff, S. 72
Bishaw, A., & Iceland, J. 14
bite marks 56-8, 107
Black women: advocacy strategies
    106-8; arrest rates 93; homicide
    rates 92; Irene's story 94-106;
    strategy use 124; use of coercive
    control 91; use of violence 89-
    92; as victim-defendants 92-4
Bohannon, J. R., Dosser, D. A., &
    Lindley, S. E. 116
Bourgois, P. 174
Brannon, R., & David, D. 187